W9-BRF-921
WITHDRAWN

Active Living Every Day

Steven N. Blair, PED
The Cooper Institute

Andrea L. Dunn, PhD
The Cooper Institute

Bess H. Marcus, PhD
Brown University Center for
Behavioral and Preventive Medicine

Ruth Ann Carpenter, MS, RD
The Cooper Institute

Peter Jaret, MA

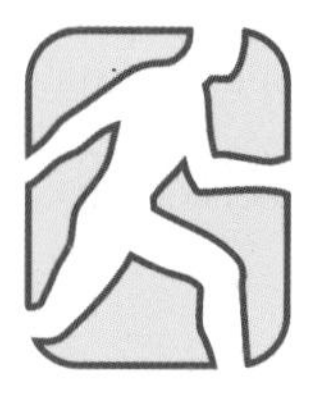

HUMAN KINETICS

Library of Congress Cataloging-in-Publication Data

Active living every day / Steven N. Blair ... [et al.].
p. cm.
Includes bibliographical references and index.
ISBN: 0-7360-3701-2
1. Exercise. 2. Physical fitness. 3. Health. I. Blair, Steven N.
RA781 .A196 2001
613.7--dc21 00-047238

ISBN: 0-7360-3701-2

Copyright @ 2001 by Steven N. Blair, Andrea L. Dunn, Bess H. Marcus, Ruth Ann Carpenter, Peter Jaret

All rights reserved. Except for use in a review, the reproduction or utilization of this work in any form or by any electronic, mechanical, or other means, now known or hereafter invented, including xerography, photocopying, and recording, and in any information storage and retrieval system, is forbidden without the written permission of the publisher.

Developmental Editor: Christine M. Drews; **Assistant Editor:** Sandra Merz Bott; **Copyeditor:** Denelle Eknes; **Proofreader:** Sarah Wiseman; **Indexer:** Craig Brown; **Permission Manager:** Courtney Astle; **Graphic Designer:** Nancy Rasmus; **Graphic Artist:** Nancy Rasmus; **Photo Manager:** Clark Brooks; **Cover Designer:** Keith Blomberg; **Photographer (cover):** Tom Roberts; **Photographers (interior):** The Terry Wild Studio: x (top), 2, 36, 64, 123, 127, 133, 153, 168; © Paul T. McMahon: x (bottom), 15; © Cheyenne Rowe/International Stock: 1; © Patrick Ramsey/International Stock: 4; © Mikeo Photography: 7, 80; © Scott Barrow/ International Stock: 10, 63, 67; © Oscar C. Williams: 13, 16, 35, 69, 99 (right), 113, 141; Tom Roberts/Human Kinetics: 18, 53, 58, 87, 117; © Dennis Light: 21, 54; © William L. Wantland/Tom Stack and Associates: 23; ; Anea/Vohra/Unicorn Stock Photos: 25; Earl Kogler/International Stock: 29; Raymond J. Malace: 30, 97, 129, 138; Martha McBride/Unicorn Stock Photos: 32; Brian Drake/ SportsChrome-USA: 39, 165; CLEO Freelance Photography: 61; Jean Higgins/Unicorn Stock Photos: 62; Dennis MacDonald/ Unicorn Stock Photos: 70; Kristen Olenick: 76; David Sanders: 79, 134, 166; Steve Wolper/Ocean Images: 88; Jim Shipper/Unicorn Stock Photos: 89; Mark Bolster/International Stock: 95; Crystal Images/Kathleen Marie Menke: 99 (left), ; Skjold Photographs: 100; Mrs. Kevin Scheibel: 107, 158; Giovanni Lundari/International Stock: 111 (left); Mark E. Gibson/The Image Finders: 111 (right), 114 (right); Bachmann/The Image Finders: 112; Michael Philip Manheim/The Image Finders: 114 (left); © W. Ron Sutton, President, Accusplit: 118, 119; Bob Jacobson/International Stock: 125; Tom Messenger: 136; Mary E. Messenger: 137; Photo by Stan Gregg: 145; Ray Goforth: 149; Joanna Gleason: 150; Action Images: 157; © S.D. Peterson: Photo of Peter Jaret, 194; **Art Manager:** Craig Newsom; **Illustrators:** Dick Flood and Roberto Sabas

Notice: Permission to reproduce the following material is granted to persons and agencies who have purchased *Active Living Every Day:* pp. 3-4, 5, 12, 17, 18, 20, 26, 27, 31, 41-42, 44-46, 48, 49, 56, 65, 67, 71-74, 75, 76, 81-82, 85, 91-92, 102-103, 104-105, 110, 115, 120, 127, 131, 135-136, 142, 143, 146, 154-155, 161-162, 162-163, 167-168, 174, 175, 176, 178, 184, 185, 186, and 187. The reproduction of other parts of this book is expressly forbidden by the above copyright notice. Persons or agencies who have not purchased *Active Living Every Day* may not reproduce any material.

Printed in Hong Kong 10 9 8 7 6 5 4 3 2 1

Human Kinetics
Web site: www.humankinetics.com

United States: Human Kinetics
P.O. Box 5076
Champaign, IL 61825-5076
800-747-4457
e-mail: humank@hkusa.com

Canada: Human Kinetics
475 Devonshire Road Unit 100
Windsor, ON N8Y 2L5
800-465-7301 (in Canada only)
e-mail: hkcan@mnsi.net

Europe: Human Kinetics, P.O. Box IW14
Leeds LS16 6TR, United Kingdom
+44 (0) 113 278 1708
e-mail: humank@hkeurope.com

Australia: Human Kinetics
57A Price Avenue
Lower Mitcham, South Australia 5062
08 8277 1555
e-mail: liahka@senet.com.au

New Zealand: Human Kinetics
P.O. Box 105-231, Auckland Central
09-523-3462
e-mail: hkp@ihug.co.nz

CONTENTS

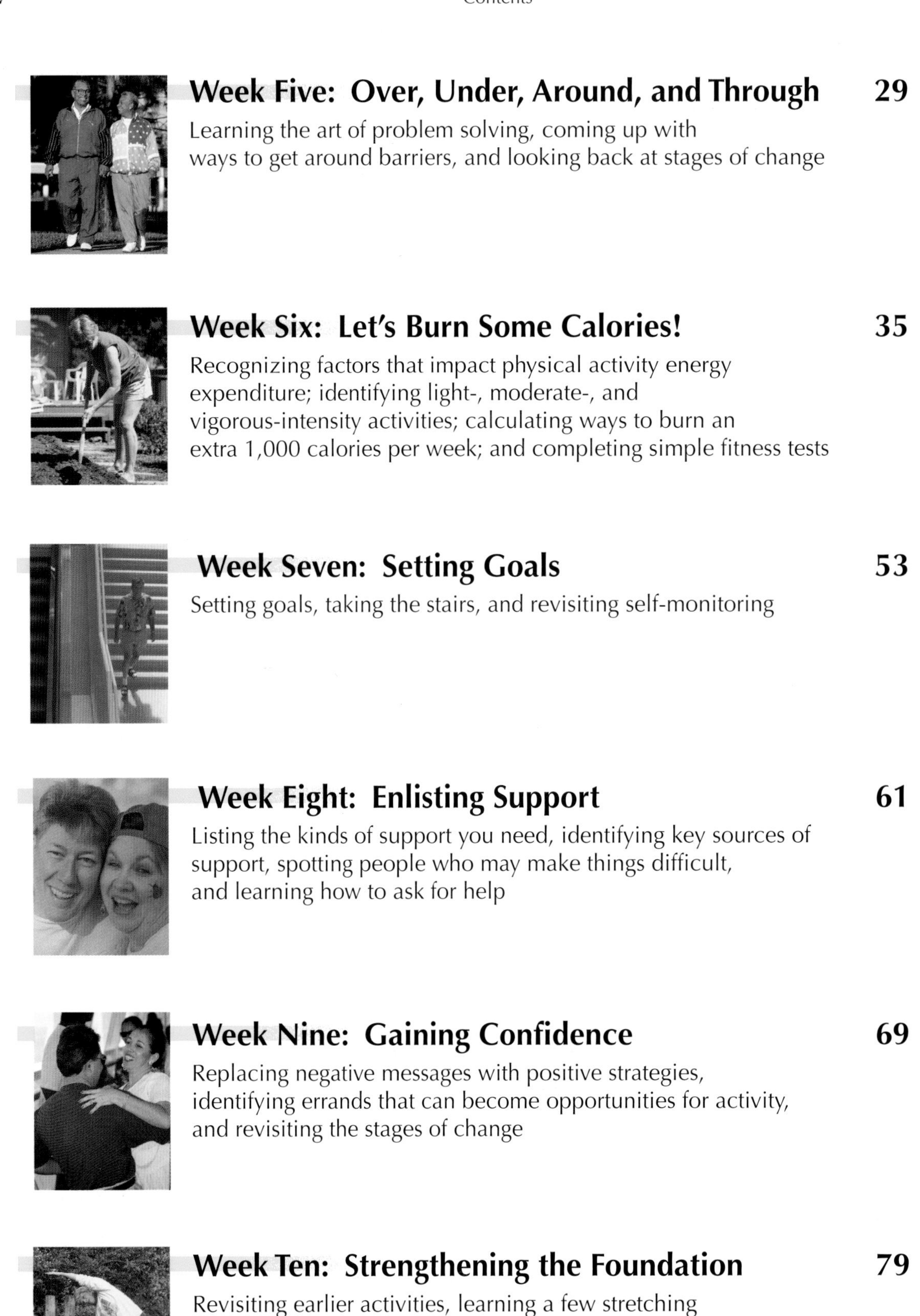

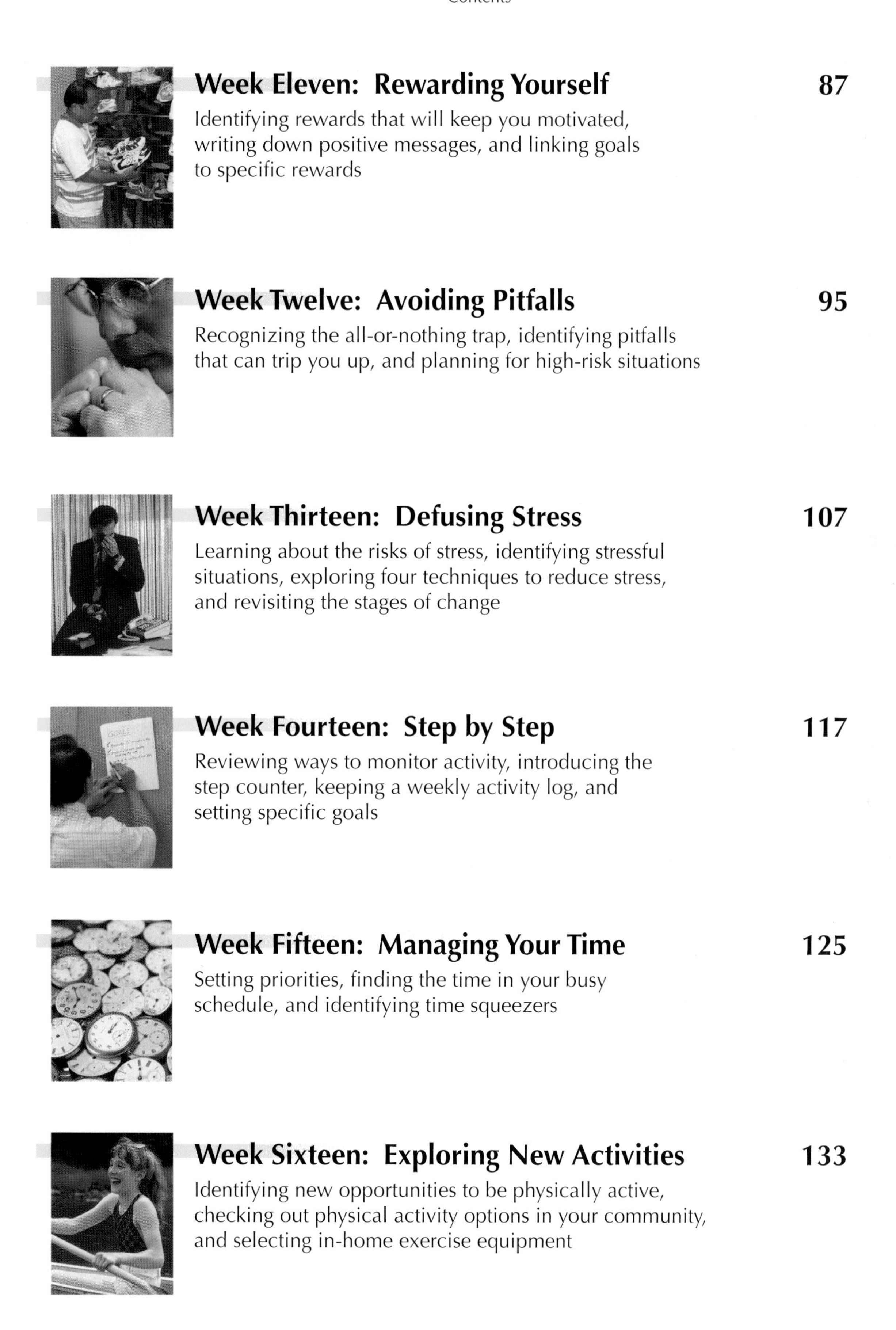

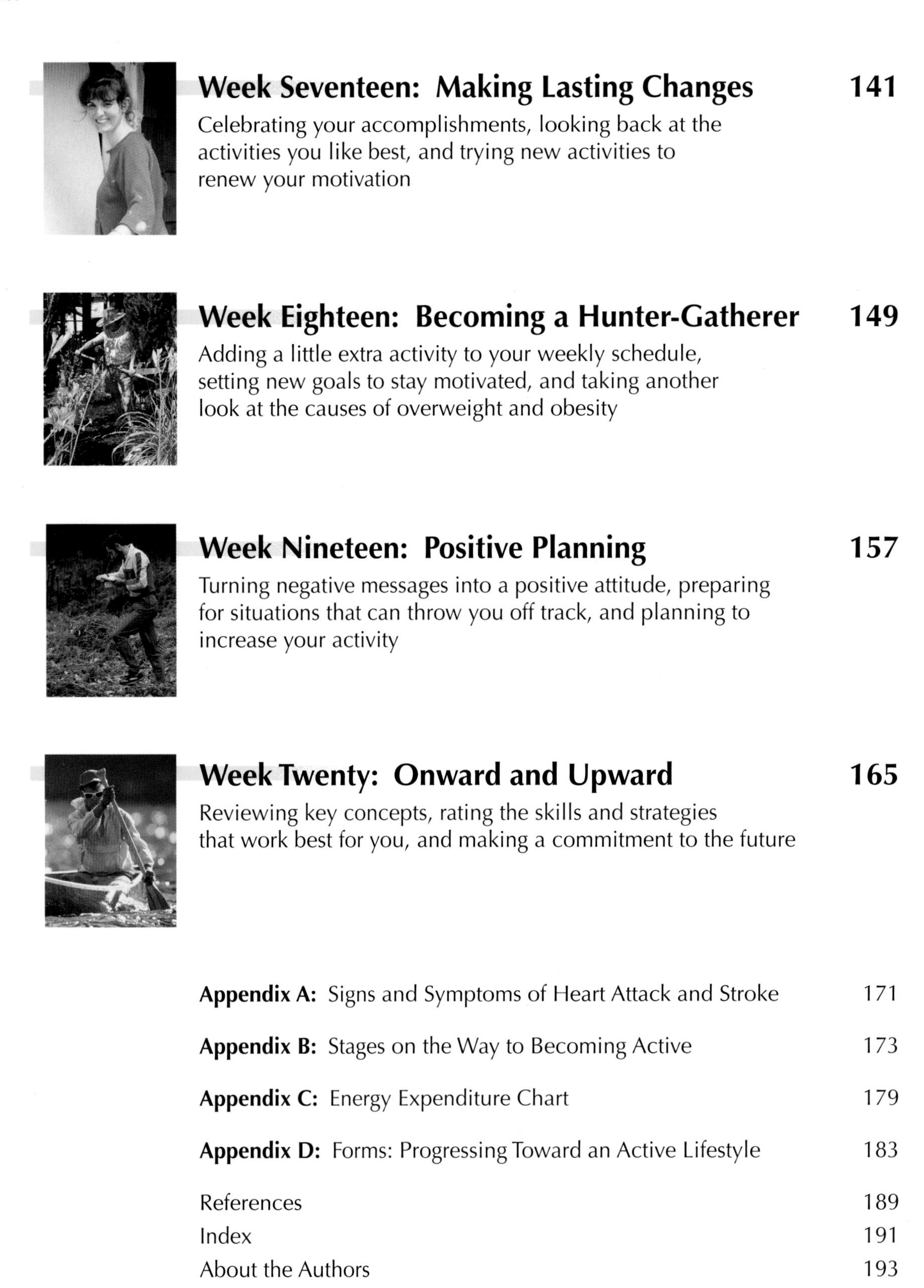

FOREWORD

For over thirty years, I have been promoting exercise as an essential component of healthy living. Maybe that's why you have picked up this book. Perhaps you want to feel healthier, have more energy, or become more fit. Maybe your doctor has told you to get more exercise or lose a little weight. You may have been unsuccessful in previous attempts to change your habits. This book could hold the key for you.

Early on, through my medical practice at The Cooper Clinic and my books, I touted the many benefits of vigorous exercise. We used to think people had to run several miles every day to stay healthy. But more recent studies have shown that even moderate amounts of exercise, like walking briskly for 30 minutes each day, can provide significant health benefits for most people.

And, as a physician, I used to think that if I told people they needed to exercise, they would do it. Many people thought all they had to do was join a gym. But becoming, and staying, active takes time, effort, and most important, the development of special lifestyle skills.

That's why I am so excited about this book. In it you will find the information, encouragement, and skill-building strategies that will help you build physical activity into your life. Top scientists at The Cooper Institute and Brown University have teamed up with a leading health writer to translate what we have tested through research into a practical, step-by-step guide. *Active Living Every Day* treats you to a state-of-the-art, proven program for improving your health and well-being through physical activity. We know that it works—people just like you have done it!

I have come a long way since the early days when I thought simply telling people to exercise at high levels was sufficient. I encourage you to take the first step to becoming active for a lifetime by diving into this book today.

To your good health,

Kenneth H. Cooper, MD, MPH
President and Founder
The Cooper Aerobics Center
Dallas, Texas

You've Come to the Right Place!

Congratulations! By opening this book, you've taken one important step toward becoming physically active. To succeed at making any change for the better, it's essential to want to change. The fact that you've come this far means you do want to change. Now all you need is a little help to make that happen.

We probably don't need to tell you that there are plenty of good reasons to add physical activity to your life. The truth is, the good news about an active lifestyle just keeps getting better. Exercise scientists and other experts have turned up a long list of benefits that come from being physically active. Nothing more strenuous than a half hour of brisk walking every day can make a big difference in your life.

Throughout the pages of this book, we'll remind you of the benefits you'll get from physical activity, but for starters, here's a quick rundown:

- Better weight control
- More energy
- Brighter mental outlook
- Increased self-esteem
- Reduced risk of heart disease, high blood pressure, and diabetes
- Reduced risk of colon cancer
- Less chance of colds and flu
- Healthy and strong bones, joints, and muscles
- Staying fit and flexible
- Living a healthier and longer independent life

Sound good? Sure it does. Let's face it, if a pill could offer so many benefits, we'd all want to take it.

Despite the good news about physical activity, most Americans still aren't active enough for their own good. According to the U.S. Surgeon General, 25 percent of adult Americans are totally sedentary, which amounts to 40 to 50 million individuals. One in four of us are bona fide couch potatoes who rarely do anything more strenuous than change channels on the TV.

There are plenty of reasons so many of us are sedentary. Hundreds of labor-saving devices, from cars and escalators to riding mowers and those

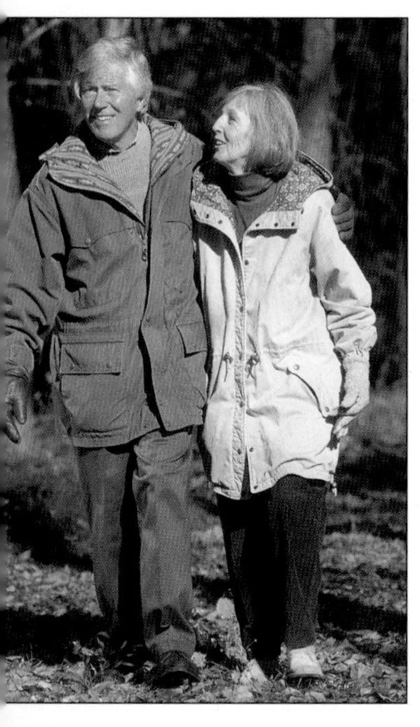

handy remote controls, have steadily taken over tasks that used to demand physical effort. These days, most jobs require us to do nothing more than sit at a desk. According to one estimate[1], most of us burn 700 to 800 fewer calories each day going about our everyday lives than people did just 25 years ago.

What can we do? One option is to find time to exercise. Some people enjoy setting aside time for a gym routine three to five times a week, but not everyone does. Many of us are already so busy with work and family that there's barely enough time in the day to do what we need to do, let alone what we know we should do.

Or so we think.

In fact, there *are* simple, easy, and enjoyable ways to add activity to your life without buying a gym membership. Walking instead of driving, dancing, riding a bike, climbing the stairs instead of taking the elevator are good ways to become active. They are also ways to incorporate activity into your everyday lifestyle, and they add up to good health, a fit body, long life, and effective weight control.

A Step-by-Step Plan That Works—And We Can Prove It

Most people don't need to be convinced that they should become active. They need to know how to do it. That's why this book is special. We've put together a step-by-step plan to help you become active every day—a plan based on scientifically tested methods.

At The Cooper Institute, we recruited 235 men and women from the Dallas area for a scientific study that we called Project *Active*. These were people who were currently doing little exercise. Half of them agreed to do a standard gym workout three to five times a week. The others were in what we called the lifestyle group. They met in small groups to talk about skills that would help them incorporate physical activities such as walking and stair climbing into their everyday lives. They also looked for other ways to boost their activity.

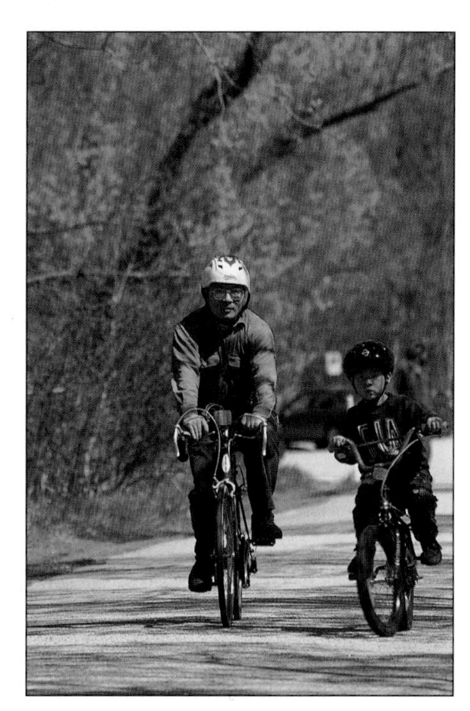

The results have been encouraging. By almost every measure, men and women in the lifestyle group enjoyed the same benefits as the people who worked out at the fitness center. After two years, their average blood pressures dropped. They lost the same amount of body fat. In fact, people in the lifestyle group were burning the same number of extra calories from activity as the hard-core gym goers and achieved the same improvements in fitness[2].

That's great news. It means you can gain virtually all the benefits of physical activity—improved weight control, healthy heart, increased energy—without signing up for a gym membership. You can make

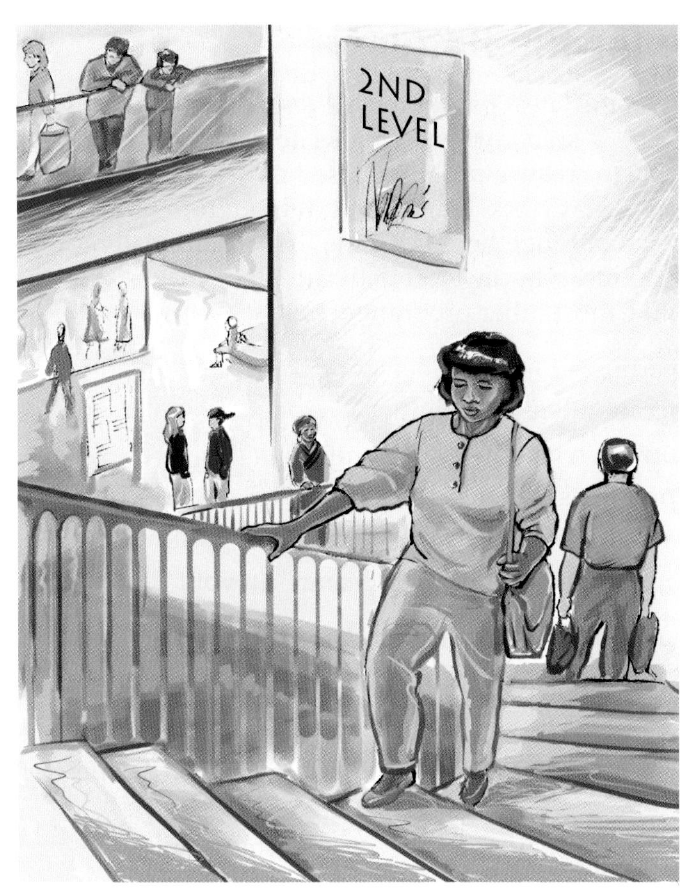

activity part of your daily life without resorting to fancy equipment or learning to love spandex. Best of all, it's a change you can live with. Two years after our program began, many participants were maintaining an active lifestyle.

How This Book Came to Be—A Little History

What led us to do the Project *Active* study? For years, beginning in the mid-1950s, exercise scientists focused almost exclusively on the health and fitness benefits of vigorous and sustained exercise. Then in 1989, findings from a study called the Aerobics Center Longitudinal Study—led by Dr. Steven Blair—helped to spark a new way of thinking about physical activity.

Men and women who were only moderately fit, the results showed, had a substantially lower risk for heart disease, stroke, and premature death than those who were unfit. People in the middle range of fitness, in fact, were half as likely to die prematurely as those in the lowest fitness category. True, the fittest people had the lowest death rates. Yet they were only 10 to 15 percent lower than people in the middle fitness group.

Don't like to go to the gym? Have we got the solution for you!

"Suddenly I started to question the advice that I and other exercise scientists were giving," Dr. Blair recalls. "When I looked at the scientific literature, I began to believe that moderate-intensity activity is enough to improve fitness and health. What really seems to matter, in terms of health and fitness, is the amount of exercise people do, not how intense the activity is."

What's more, the new evidence showed that the benefits of being moderately fit apply to almost everyone: smokers and nonsmokers, those with high cholesterol or blood pressure, even those with a family history of early cardiovascular disease. We have even found that obese individuals who are moderately fit have lower death rates than thin people who are unfit. Anyone who is sedentary and unfit can benefit enormously from becoming just moderately fit through physical activity.

That epiphany led our research group to design the study that became Project *Active*. We wanted to scientifically test the notion that people can improve their fitness and health by doing moderate-intensity everyday activities. As we've told you, the results confirmed our hunch. Moderate-intensity physical activity really does offer most of the health rewards of more vigorous exercise.

The purpose of this book, *Active Living Every Day*, is to make our lifestyle exercise program available to people everywhere. For more information about this program, please contact Human Kinetics.

Making a Change for the Better

We've based our book on the latest psychological research about behavior change, and we've gone a step further. Thanks to feedback from our volunteers, we were able to create a program based on what people need, want, and enjoy. We saw what worked and what didn't. From our participants' experiences, we've put together one of the first scientifically tested programs for increasing lifestyle physical activity. What makes our approach so special? Unlike most other programs, ours

- considers your readiness to change behavior,
- emphasizes moderate-intensity activities,
- lets you create your own activity plan,
- helps you solve problems and overcome obstacles,
- concentrates on activities you can add to your daily routine, and
- gives you tips for making other healthy changes in your life.

We're convinced that adding physical activity to everyday life is important for just about everyone. Our approach may be just what you need if

- you're not the gym type but you want to get the benefits of exercise,
- you go to the gym now and then but want more opportunities for activity,
- you want to know more about the benefits of exercise, and
- you know you should be getting more exercise but don't know how.

How to Use This Book

Making lifelong changes takes time and commitment, but it can happen. Before you get started, a few simple tips can help you get the most out of this book.

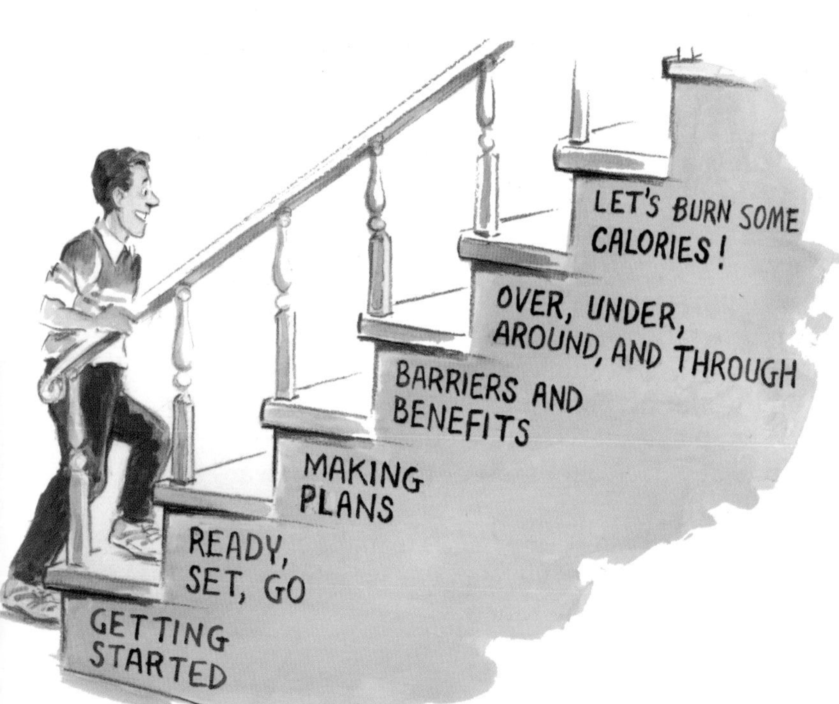

1. Take One Step at a Time

We've organized our program into 20 chapters. Each one represents a step toward increasing your physical activity. You may be tempted to rush in and make big changes all at once, especially when you've made up your mind to become more active than you have been, or you may think some steps seem too simple. Many of our participants thought the same thing at first, but as they progressed, they discovered that each step was important in the path to an active lifestyle. In fact, plenty of studies have shown that the best way for most of us to make lasting changes is one step at a time, experimenting until we find what works for us. That's why we encourage you to follow the steps in each chapter.

2. Go at Your Own Pace

We designed this book for you to go through one chapter each week, but you may go through one chapter quickly and another more slowly. That's fine. The important thing is to make a deal with yourself at the start to go through each chapter completely. As you increase your everyday physical activities, you may find you want to do more. For example, you may want to go for a longer walk than you have done before, or you may want to do something more vigorous than a walk. Go for it. The more you do, the better off you'll be, and if you bog down and need a refresher, feel free to skip back to a previous week. Our volunteers often found that they learned something new or improved their understanding by reviewing material from earlier in the program.

3. Track Your Progress

Throughout this book, we'll be asking you to write down information. It's important to keep track of your progress so you'll know where you started and what you've achieved. (We've included forms to make it easier.) You may also want to buy a pocket-sized spiral notebook to keep with you during the day so you don't have to lug us around. That way you can record your activities or ideas and write them in your notebook. Later we'll talk about step counters—a nifty device that can help you track your progress. For many of our participants, step counters were tremendously helpful.

Along the way, we've added signposts to make this book simple to use:

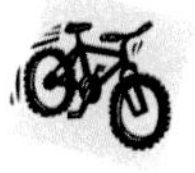

Activity Alerts spotlight the activities we'd like you to do in each chapter.

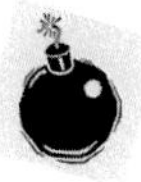

Myth Busters debunk some common misconceptions about physical activity and lifestyle changes—misconceptions that get in the way of you becoming active.

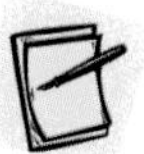

Expert Advice offers tips we learned from administering the lifestyle programs at The Cooper Institute and Brown University as well as some findings from other research centers—information that can help you become active.

Up Close and Personal offers composite sketches of people who have successfully adopted active lifestyles.

Did You Know? offers surprising facts about physical activity and its benefits, many of which include the latest research findings from labs around the world.

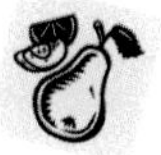

Weighing In highlights advice for people interested in achieving a healthy weight.

Congratulations on picking up this book. We are confident that you can become active, fit, and healthy and that this book can give you the motivation you need. We're looking forward to helping you become active every day.

WEEK **ONE**

Getting Started

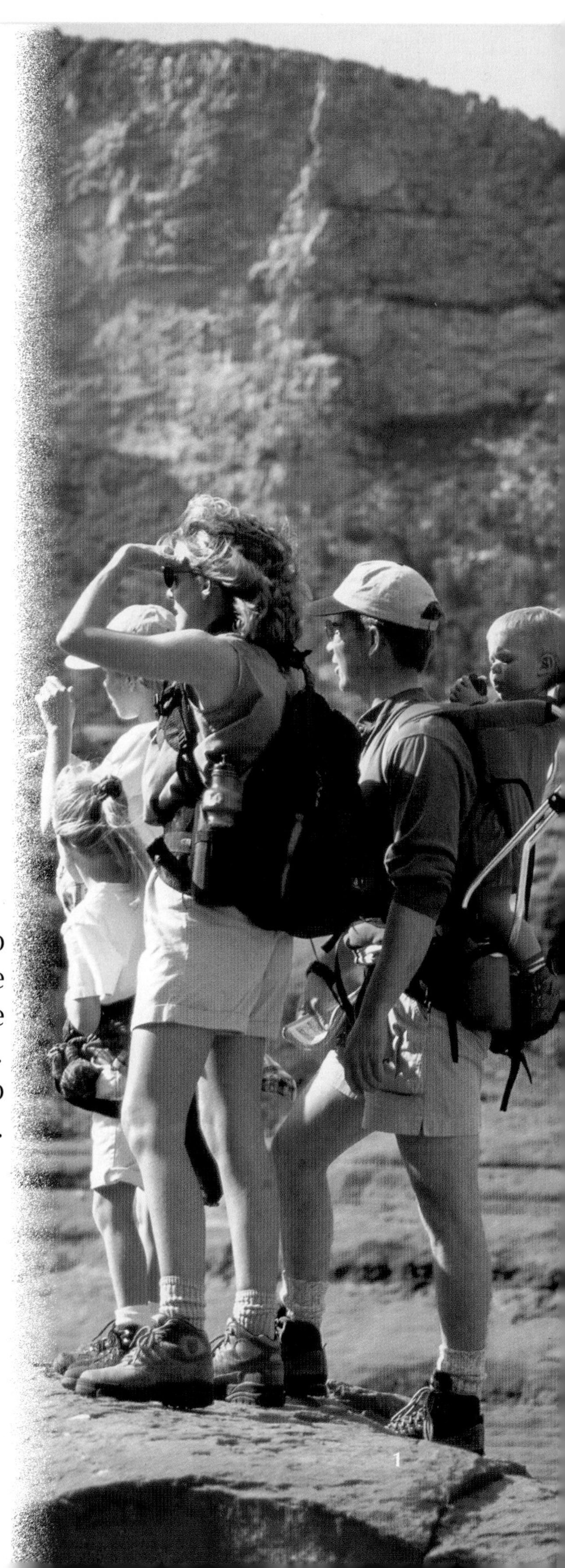

In This Chapter

- Thinking about successful habit changes
- Assessing the need to see a doctor before increasing activity

So here you are, ready to get active, but how do you do that? Where do you start? Don't worry. We will show you the way. First, let's look at three people who have used the Active Living program. Two of them have turned their sedentary lives into full, active lives and one has not, at least, not yet. Can you spot why?

Yolanda has been pretty sedentary since high school. She is busy working full time and being a single mom to two young children. This doesn't leave a lot of time for exercise, but Yolanda learned in the Active Living program that she doesn't have to do all her exercise at once to get health benefits. This freed her to think about the brief segments of time she has at work each day when she can fit in 5 or 10 minutes of walking. A few coworkers walk with her on Tuesdays and Thursdays, which helps keep her going when she doesn't feel like it. As her fitness has improved, she has added stairs to her walking routine. After 13 months, Yolanda now does 30 to 45 minutes of activity at work at least four days a week and does some physical activity with her kids on one day of the weekend.

Tommy was on several varsity teams in high school, but he stopped playing sports because the community college he went to didn't have athletic teams. As a building supplies salesperson, he spends a lot of time in the car going from job site to job site. Occasionally he plays a pick-up game of basketball, but frequent knee injuries have kept him sidelined a lot. Tommy joined the Active Living program at his doctor's recommendation. He was reluctant at first because it didn't seem tough enough. He thought he should work up a big sweat, strain hard, and have sore muscles, but he learned that doing moderate-intensity activities was a good place for him to start. He made a list of the benefits of getting active and used goal-setting strategies to help him stay on track. One important skill Tommy learned was to think ahead about situations (e.g., injuries, work crises, family time commitments) that might sidetrack his physical activity. He then planned alternative strategies such as cycling instead of running when he was injured, walking five minutes at each job site when he couldn't fit in a regular workout, and finding ways to enjoy his family and be active at the same time. Now regularly active, Tommy has fewer knee injuries and a lot more energy than before he participated in the Active Living program.

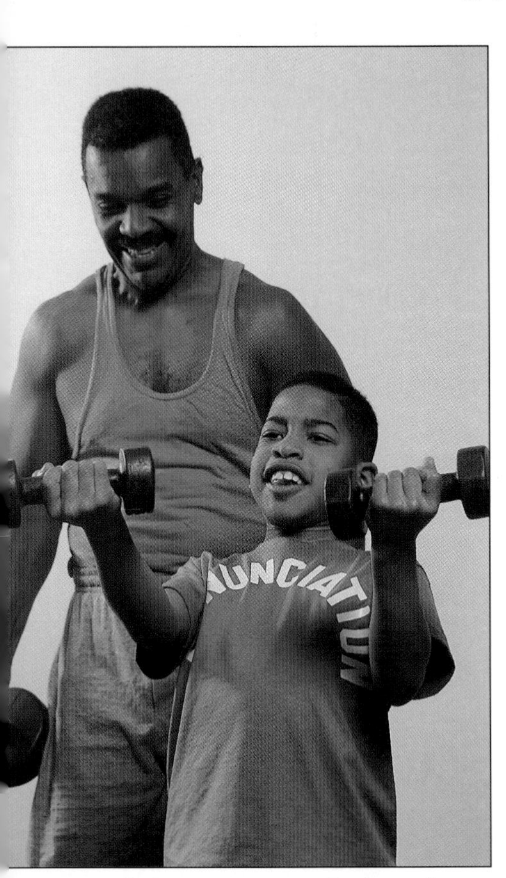

We will show you ways to fit physical activity into your everyday life.

Gwen started the program with the primary intent to lose weight. She had gained 18 pounds since her wedding 14 years ago and was eager to get it off. She had tried all the miracle cures and fad diets, with short-term success and long-term regrets. She heard about the Active Living program from a friend. She was aware of how to cut calories and fat, but she wanted to increase her activity level. She got frustrated early on when she didn't lose a lot of weight quickly. Also, she didn't like keeping track of her daily physical activity or completing the tasks in each of the Active Living program chapters. However, she kept coming to the weekly group sessions. She learned about the benefits other than weight loss that some people were getting as they increased their activity. She also learned that there was no quick fix to changing her activity level. It took time, energy, commitment, and most of all, developing lifestyle management skills. At the end of six months, Gwen was not any more active than when she started, but she is more ready to try some new strategies she learned from the Active Living program. So she is going to go through the book again on her own.

Like Gwen, we all have goals we want to achieve. And like Yolanda and Tommy, we need to learn specific skills and strategies that can help us achieve our goals. For Yolanda, it took getting her physical activities in short bouts during her workday. Tommy found that gradually building up his physical activity and planning for high-risk situations helped him achieve his goal of getting fit and having more energy than he had before he started. What will it be for you? This book will help you identify ways you can succeed in living an active life every day. Let's start by looking at habits you have already changed for the better.

ACTIVITY ALERT

What Habits Have You Changed?

Like most people, you've probably made changes in the way you live. Maybe you've quit smoking or cut back on the fat in your diet. Maybe you've started a new hobby or signed up for a course at the community college. Even small changes, such as fastening your seatbelt every time you get in the car, are important, even lifesaving. They prove that you can change your habits for the better.

MY PERSONAL SUCCESSES — HABITS I'VE CHANGED FOR THE BETTER

Take a few minutes now to list one or more of your personal success stories—unwanted habits you've dropped or good ones you've adopted. Many people have given up smoking, for instance, or stopped biting their fingernails. Many of us have switched from whole milk to 2 percent, or even skim. We've learned to cook low-fat meals and choose more fruits and vegetables at the grocery store.

Think about why you were able to make a successful change, even a small one. What helped you succeed? What got in your way? Maybe the biggest obstacle for you was having enough time, or getting distracted during the holiday, or losing your determination. Think about two or three habits you've changed and fill in the following form.

Habits I've changed

1. ______________________________

2. ______________________________

3. ______________________________

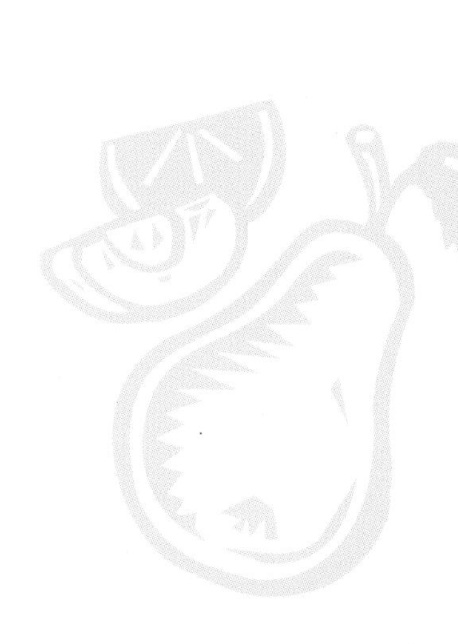

(continued)

(continued)

Things that helped me succeed

1. ____________________

2. ____________________

3. ____________________

Obstacles that got in my way

1. ____________________

2. ____________________

3. ____________________

Are you impressed with yourself? We hope so. Changing habits is difficult, but look at the ones you have already successfully changed! You can do the same thing with physical activity. We know you can! Later in this book, we'll look at strategies for long-term success and simple ways to sidestep obstacles.

? DID YOU KNOW?

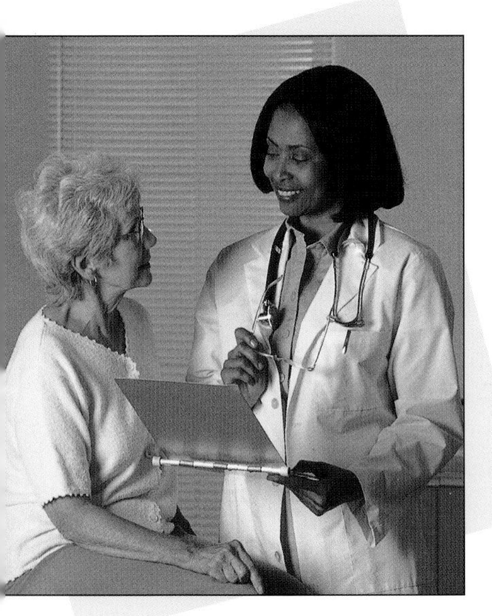

Moderate-intensity activity is equivalent to a brisk walk. How brisk is brisk? If you're walking at a moderate-intensity pace, you should complete a mile (1.6 km) in 15 to 20 minutes. Research studies by us and others have shown that at least 30 minutes of any moderately intense physical activity every day will improve your health and function.

Do I Need a Medical Exam?

In general, exercising at a moderate intensity is safe for most people. One great advantage of becoming more active through moderate-intensity physical activities is that for most people, a medical exam or stress test is not required before increasing activity. Still, some people who have preexisting diseases, such as heart disease and diabetes, should check with their doctors before beginning to exercise at a moderate intensity. Use the following questionnaire to help you decide if you should check with your doctor.

ACTIVITY ALERT

Should I See My Doctor?

Please read the PAR-Q & You questionnaire carefully and answer each question honestly. Check yes or no next to each question.

The questionnaire will help you determine if you are ready to become more physically active. If you answered yes to one or more questions, talk with your doctor before you increase your physical activity. Be sure to tell your doctor about the questions to which you answered yes.

If you answered no to all questions, you can increase your activity by beginning slowly and building up gradually—just as we show you in this book. Periodically review this questionnaire and contact your doctor if you answer yes to any of the questions.

Physical Activity Readiness Questionnaire – PAR-Q (revised 1994)

PAR - Q & YOU

(A Questionnaire for People Aged 15 to 69)

Regular physical activity is fun and healthy, and increasingly more people are starting to become more active every day. Being more active is very safe for most people. However, some people should check with their doctor before they start becoming much more physically active.

If you are planning to become much more physically active than you are now, start by answering the seven questions in the box below. If you are between the ages of 15 and 69, the PAR-Q will tell you if you should check with your doctor before you start. If you are over 69 years of age, and you are not used to being very active, check with your doctor.

Common sense is your best guide when you answer these questions. Please read the questions carefully and answer each one honestly: check YES or NO.

YES	NO	
☐	☐	1. Has your doctor ever said that you have a heart condition and that you should only do physical activity recommended by a doctor?
☐	☐	2. Do you feel pain in your chest when you do physical activity?
☐	☐	3. In the past month, have you had chest pain when you were not doing physical activity?
☐	☐	4. Do you lose your balance because of dizziness or do you ever lose consciousness?
☐	☐	5. Do you have a bone or joint problem that could be made worse by a change in your physical activity?
☐	☐	6. Is your doctor currently prescribing drugs (for example, water pills) for your blood pressure or heart condition?
☐	☐	7. Do you know of any other reason why you should not do physical activity?

If you answered

YES to one or more questions

Talk with your doctor by phone or in person BEFORE you start becoming much more physically active or BEFORE you have a fitness appraisal. Tell your doctor about the PAR-Q and which questions you answered YES.

- You may be able to do any activity you want—as long as you start slowly and build up gradually. Or, you may need to restrict your activities to those which are safe for you. Talk with your doctor about the kinds of activities you wish to participate in and follow his/her advice.
- Find out which community programs are safe and helpful for you.

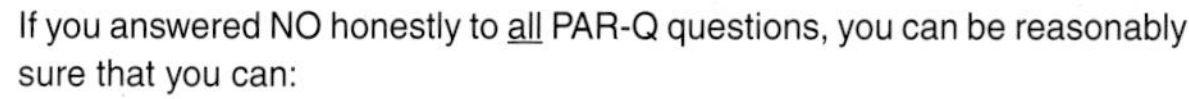

If you answered NO honestly to all PAR-Q questions, you can be reasonably sure that you can:

- start becoming much more physically active—begin slowly and build up gradually. This is the safest and easiest way to go.
- take part in a fitness appraisal—this is an excellent way to determine your basic fitness so that you can plan the best way for you to live actively.

DELAY BECOMING MUCH MORE ACTIVE:

- if you are not feeling well because of a temporary illness such as a cold or a fever—wait until you feel better; or
- if you are or may be pregnant—talk to your doctor before you start becoming more active.

Please note: If your health changes so that you then answer YES to any of the above questions, tell your fitness or health professional. Ask whether you should change your physical activity plan.

Informed Use of the PAR-Q: The Canadian Society for Exercise Physiology, Health Canada, and their agents assume no liability for persons who undertake physical activity, and if in doubt after completing this questionnaire, consult your doctor prior to physical activity.

You are encouraged to copy the PAR-Q but only if you use the entire form

NOTE: If the PAR-Q is being given to a person before he or she participates in a physical activity program or a fitness appraisal, this section may be used for legal or administrative purposes.

I have read, understood and completed this questionnaire. Any questions I had were answered to my full satisfaction.

NAME ______________________

SIGNATURE ______________________ DATE ______________________

SIGNATURE OF PARENT ______________________ WITNESS ______________________
or GUARDIAN (for participants under the age of majority)

©Canadian Society for Exercise Physiology
Société canadienne de physiologie de l'exercice

Supported by: 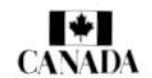

Health Canada Santé Canada

If you are starting with this book, chances are you are pretty sedentary and should begin doing moderate-intensity activities. However, if you want to exercise at a vigorous level, check with your doctor first if you

1. are a man 45 or older or a woman 55 or older; *or*
2. have *two* or more of the following risk factors: family history of heart disease, are currently a cigarette smoker, have high blood pressure, high cholesterol, high blood sugar, are at least 30 pounds (13.6 kg) overweight, or are currently not at all active; *or*
3. have heart or blood vessel disease, diabetes, lung disease, asthma, thyroid disorders, or kidney disease.

? DID YOU KNOW?

Whether or not you need to check with your doctor before going any further with the Active Living program, you should know the warning signs of a heart attack or stroke. No, we don't expect you to have a heart attack during this program. In fact, you'll learn how activity *reduces* your risk for heart disease along with other health problems. But, being able to identify the warning signs will not only help *you*, it will also prepare you to help friends and loved ones if they ever suffer a heart attack or stroke. For more information, review appendix A.

Like Yolanda and Tommy at the beginning of this chapter, we hope you will change your life for the better by working through this program. We know you can do it, because you have already been successful in changing other habits. Each week, we will provide you with a reminder of what we hope you accomplish that week. Here's the first one:

Chapter Checklist

Before you move on to the next week's activities, make sure you

- Identified at least one habit you have successfully changed
- Completed the PAR-Q & You questionnaire and, if necessary, made an appointment to talk with or visit your doctor for clearance to increase your physical activity level
- Memorized the warning signs of a heart attack and stroke

This week you read about two people who have worked through the Active Living program and changed their lives for the better, you have looked at your own successes in changing habits, and you have made sure you are medically ready to participate in this program. Now we're ready to dive in. Let's get to it. Week 2, here we come!

WEEK **TWO**

Ready, Set, Go

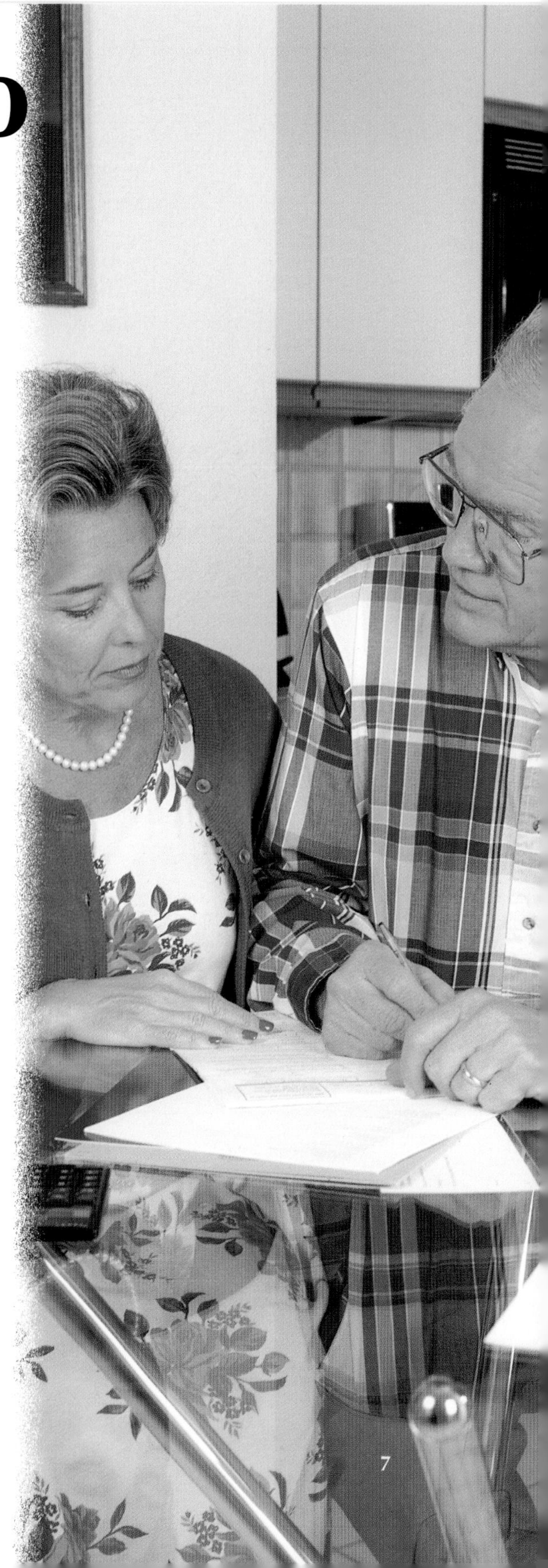

In This Chapter

- Identifying your readiness for change
- Conducting your Personal Time Study
- Weighing the weight-loss benefits of activity
- Finding time to get up and move

Ready to get moving? That's great. The purpose of this second week is to identify opportunities when you can turn inactivity into activity, but first we'd like to talk about how people change.

EXPERT ADVICE

Making a Change

We've all made New Year's resolutions to lose weight or begin exercising, and perhaps we've even stuck with them for a while. Too often, life gets in the way, and we watch our best intentions fall apart.

Why? Change doesn't happen all at once, and not all of us begin at the same starting point. Researchers have identified five stages of change that most people go through along the way to adopting new habits and behaviors. They are

1. precontemplation (not even thinking about it),
2. contemplation (giving it a thought now and then, but not doing it),
3. preparation (doing it irregularly),
4. action (doing the new habit consistently but for less than six months), and
5. maintenance (maintaining the new habit for six months or more).

The point is, change takes place in stages, and progress isn't always in one direction. For every two giant steps forward there may be one step back. That's normal. Every move, forward or back, is part of the normal process of habit change. You may stay in the stage of contemplation for a long time before you move forward, or you may go through the stage of preparation quickly, then stay in action for a short time, stumble, and end up back in contemplation or preparation for a while. This isn't a sign of failure. It's a sign that you're trying to change.

What's the key to moving through the stages? Using special skills such as keeping track of your progress, recruiting help, removing barriers, preventing lapses, and thinking positively. Studies at Brown University show that learning these skills really helps people increase their physical activity levels. This book is designed to help you learn and practice these and other helpful strategies to become physically active for a lifetime.

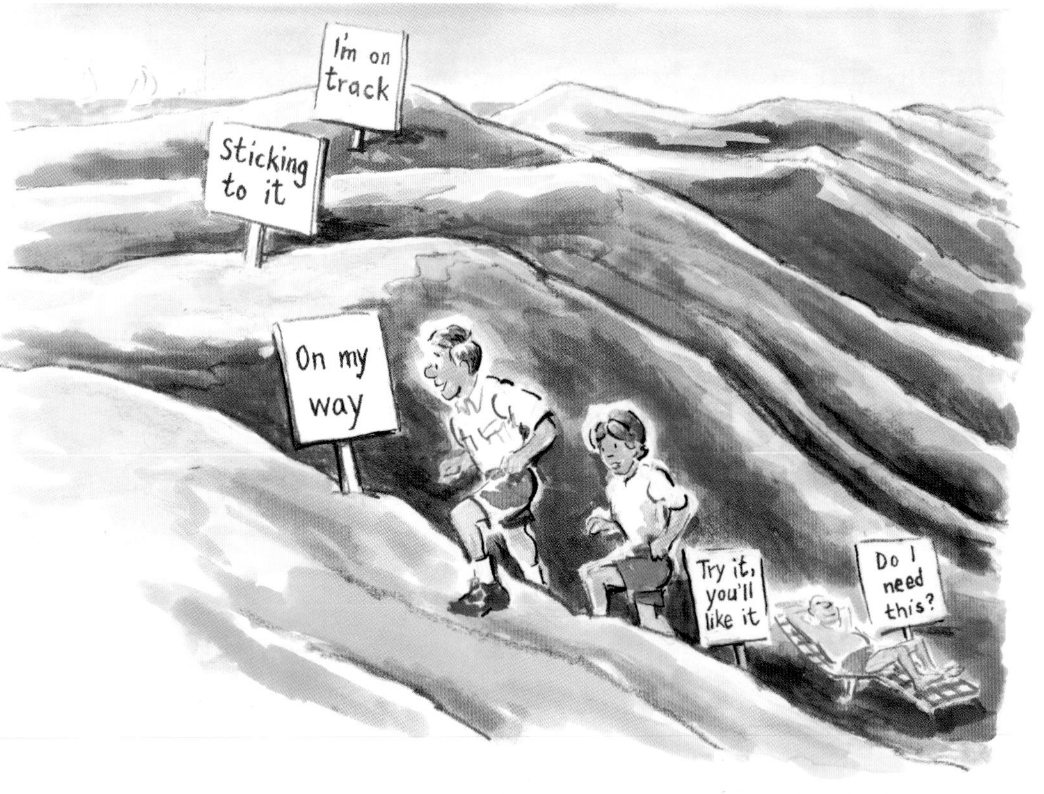

ACTIVITY ALERT

Identifying Your Readiness to Change

So let's see where you are right now. Knowing your stage of change can help you discover what you need to do to move forward. The following questions will help you gauge how ready you are to change. In the coming weeks, we'll return to this flow chart to track your progress, so be honest in your answers.

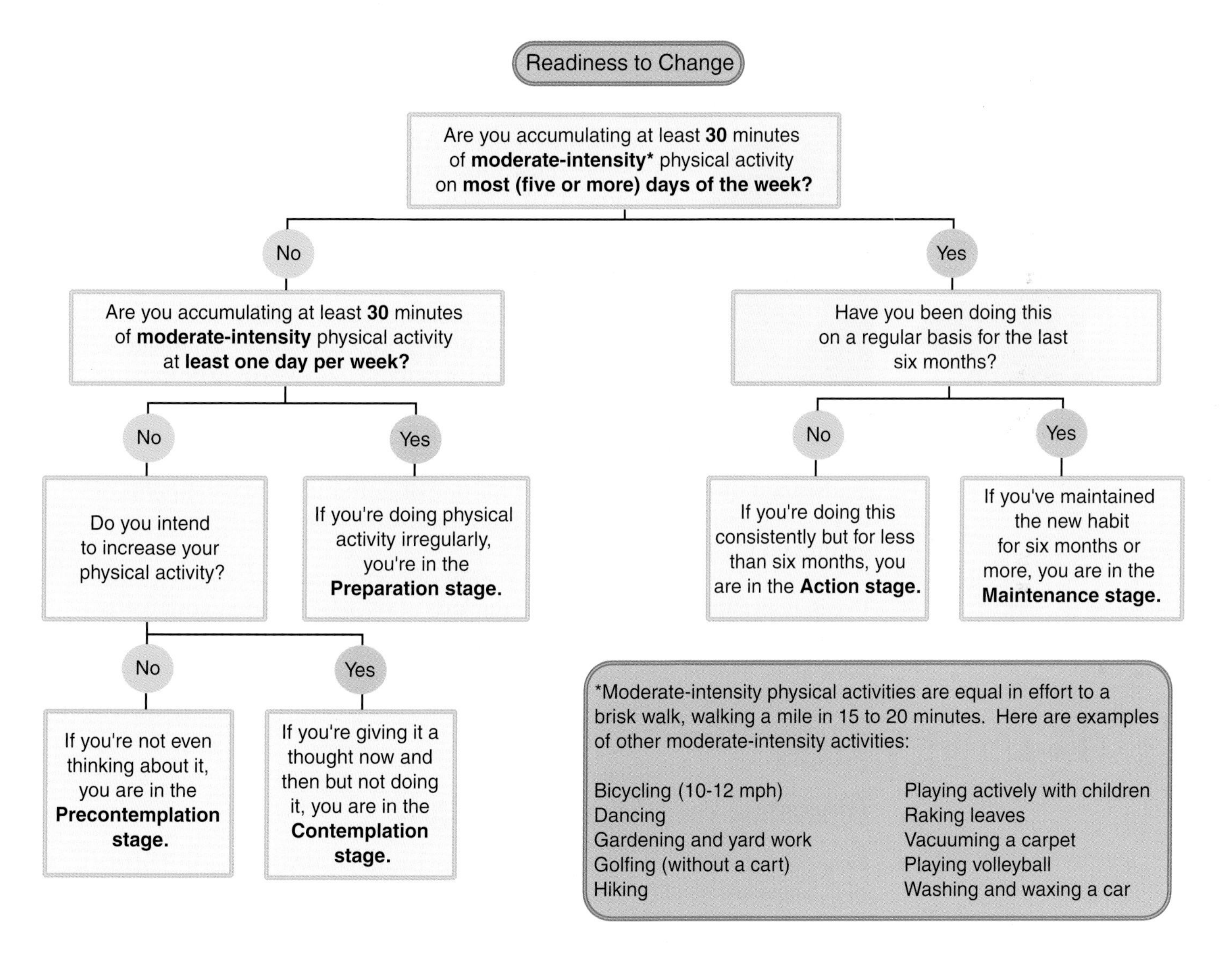

EXPERT ADVICE

Let's say you find yourself in the precontemplation stage—you are not even thinking about exercise. What's next? Check appendix B, where you'll find handy references with advice targeted to each stage. For example, "Do I Need This?" (page 173) contains advice for precontemplators, including many reasons to become active. If you're contemplating becoming active, check out "Try It, You'll Like It" on page 175. If you find yourself in preparation, look at "On My Way" (page 175), where you'll find great tips on overcoming obstacles. If you're in the action stage, see page 176, and if you're in the maintenance stage see page 177. Several research studies at Brown University have shown that these handy references help people change successfully.

Finding Opportunities to Get Up and Move

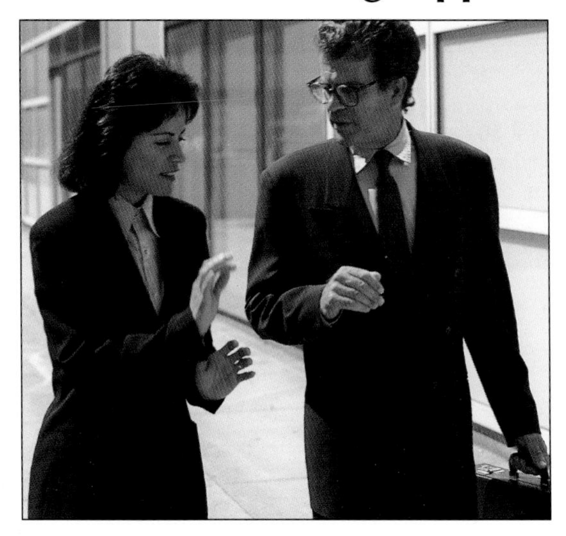

What's one of the biggest roadblocks to an active lifestyle? The chair. Another obstacle is thinking that you'd like to exercise but you don't have the time. Why are so many Americans overweight? In large part because most of us don't get up and move often enough. We sit in waiting rooms, we sit at the airport terminal, and we sit in our cars. Of course, there are times when we can't help but sit—at our desks or in a movie theater, for instance.

But, there *are* plenty of other times when we're in waiting rooms, or airport terminals, or even watching the kids' soccer games when we could be moving around instead of sitting. One marketing manager we know at Apple Computer conducts her one-on-one meetings on foot, walking around the company's landscaped grounds. A volunteer for one of our studies made a point of hitting the mute button on her television during the commercials and getting up to do something active.

The point is simple: There are plenty of opportunities for activity, between television shows, watching the kids play soccer, during your coffee break, or while you're waiting for the oven to heat up. The first trick is to find them. The second is to take advantage of them.

ACTIVITY ALERT

Conducting Your Personal Time Study

How do you spend your time? Most of us have a rough idea, of course, but few of us know where all those minutes go in our crowded lives. So we're going to ask you to take a close look at how you spend your time. The reason is simple. By looking at how you spend your time, you'll identify opportunities for activity you might not have known existed.

First, select one typical weekday and one typical weekend day over the next week. Mark them both on your calendar.

Then, use the Personal Time Study sheet you'll find on page 184. Fill it in, recording your activities in four-hour blocks. (Some people like to record their daily routines in one-hour blocks to get a detailed picture of how they spend their time. That's fine. You can use a notepad to break down the time however you like.)

After you've recorded your activities, determine how many minutes you spend doing any type of physical activity and how many minutes you are inactive—sitting, sleeping, driving a car, watching television, or talking on the phone, for instance.

Throughout this book, as you'll see, we provide many worksheets like this. Feel free to photocopy them for your use. For instance, we want you to fill out a time sheet for one weekday and another for a weekend day. A few of the forms you will use most often appear again in appendix D. You can use all the worksheets for activities you would like to return to when you're struggling to find time to stick to your plan, for instance, or when problems at home or work may be threatening to knock you off track. You might also want to do this with a friend, then compare notes on how you spend your days.

Here's what a sample entry might look like:

Example

Date: ________________ Day of week: ______________________

Time slot	Tasks/activities	Physically active? Yes	No
8:00 A.M. to noon	Desk work:		75 minutes
	Meeting:		120 minutes
	Walk to and from car:	7 minutes	
	Walk to vending machine:	3 minutes	
	Walk to meeting:	4 minutes	
	Talk with coworkers:		31 minutes
	Total time	**14 min.**	**226 min.**
Noon to 4:00 P.M.	Walk to lunch room:	5 minutes	
	Lunch:		30 minutes
	Walk back to office:	5 minutes	
	Desk work:		180 minutes
	Walk to lunch room:	5 minutes	
	Coffee break:		10 minutes
	Return to office:	5 minutes	
	Total time	**20 min.**	**220 min.**

PERSONAL TIME STUDY

Record your activities for one weekday and one weekend day. Use one sheet for each day. Try to keep this page, or a notepad if you prefer, with you and write things down as you go. Remember to add up the minutes you were physically active and record those in the "Yes" column. Then add up the minutes you were inactive. The total active and inactive for each four-hour block should be 240 minutes. Add up the total number of active and inactive minutes in your day at the bottom of the sheet.

(continued)

(continued)

Date: ____________________ Day of week: ________________________

Time slot	Tasks/activities	Physically active? Yes	No
Midnight to 4:00 A.M.			
4:01 to 8:00 A.M.			
8:01 A.M. to noon			
12:01 to 4:00 P.M.			
4:01 to 8:00 P.M.			
8:01 P.M. to midnight			
	Total time		

Surprised by how much time you spend sitting? You're not alone. The modern world, with all its conveniences, has conspired to make life inactive for most of us. It doesn't have to be that way. That's why the Personal Time Study is so useful. Many of the minutes when you're now inactive are golden opportunities to become active.

UP CLOSE & PERSONAL

Jorge didn't think of himself as a couch dweller. Sure, he liked to relax at the end of a long day, but he never realized how much time he spent sitting until he completed a Personal Time Study. There it was, in black and white: almost every waking hour he spent either sitting on the bus, sitting at his desk at work, returning on the bus, or sitting down to read a newspaper or watch TV. Looking over what he did every day, or rather, how little he did in the way of physical activity, sounded the alarm for him and made him serious about turning some of that downtime into activity. It also reminded him of something: before he and his wife had kids and his job became so hectic, he used to walk instead of drive to the commuter bus stop. Maybe now, he began to think, would be a good time to get back into that habit.

WEIGHING IN

A Word About Weight Control

To Lose a Little Weight

- Eat 500 fewer calories each day, *or*
- Burn 500 extra calories each day, *or*
- Do a little of both—reduce calorie intake by 250 a day and increase energy expenditure by 250 calories a day.

These days, Americans are obsessed with weight loss. We spend tens of billions of dollars a year on diets and weight-loss plans. Yet obesity is rapidly increasing. What we've learned is that dieting alone doesn't work for most people. Even dieters who lose weight typically gain it back. Dozens of studies have shown that the people who reliably lose weight and keep it off are those who slightly decrease the calories they eat *and* increase the calories they burn through physical activity.

There may be a special advantage to exercise when it comes to losing weight and keeping it off for good. You don't have to cut back so much on your daily calories. Here's why. It takes a 500-calorie-per-day deficit to lose one pound of body fat per week. You can do this by

- eating 500 calories less per day,
- eating 250 calories less and increasing your physical activity by 250 calories per day, or
- increasing your physical activity by 500 calories per day.

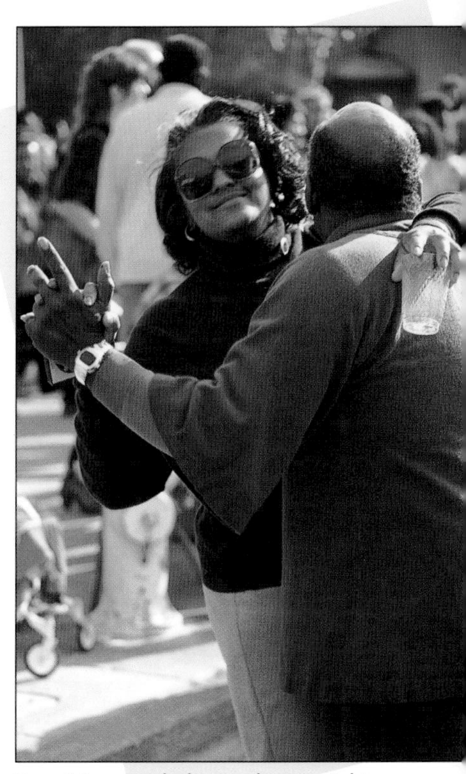
Exercising can help you lose weight and keep it off.

The second and third options not only give you the added bonus of all the different health benefits from exercise but you get to eat more than in the first option. Being able to eat more increases the likelihood you will get more of the important nutrients.

Not everyone starts off enjoying physical activity, of course. For some people it seems like slow torture at first. If that sounds like you, don't despair. We'll help you find ways to fit in three easy 10-minute walks during the day that offer most of the benefits of more extended activity. We'll even try to make it fun. For almost everyone, it's easier to say "yes" three times a day to a brisk walk than "no" many times a day to food.

Don't get us wrong: A healthy diet is important, but the best way to lose weight and keep it off, we think, is to increase your activity every day and make activity a lifelong habit.

UP CLOSE & PERSONAL

Remember Jorge? He wasn't the only one in his family to understand how sedentary he had become. Intrigued by the Personal Time Study, his wife Teresa filled one out for herself. With three kids to look after and an office job, she felt as if she never stopped. But when she took a closer look she realized that she spent most of her time sitting—in the car while driving the kids here and there, at her desk and in meetings, watching the kids at dance practice or piano recitals. About the only time she got up and moved, she realized, was when she was preparing meals. *That*, she decided then and there, was going to have to change.

EXPERT ADVICE

In our programs at The Cooper Institute and Brown University, we have helped many people identify their readiness to change. We always ask participants how long they have been thinking about increasing their activity. The record? Thirty years! That participant went on to become one of the stars of our program. The moral of the story: it's never too late to get started.

Chapter Checklist

Before you move on to the next week's activities, make sure you

- Filled out the Readiness to Change form
- Completed a Personal Time Study for two days
- Identified opportunities during the day to add physical activity

Now you have a better idea of where all the time in your day goes. In the next week, we'll look at how to turn inactivity into activity.

WEEK THREE

Making Plans

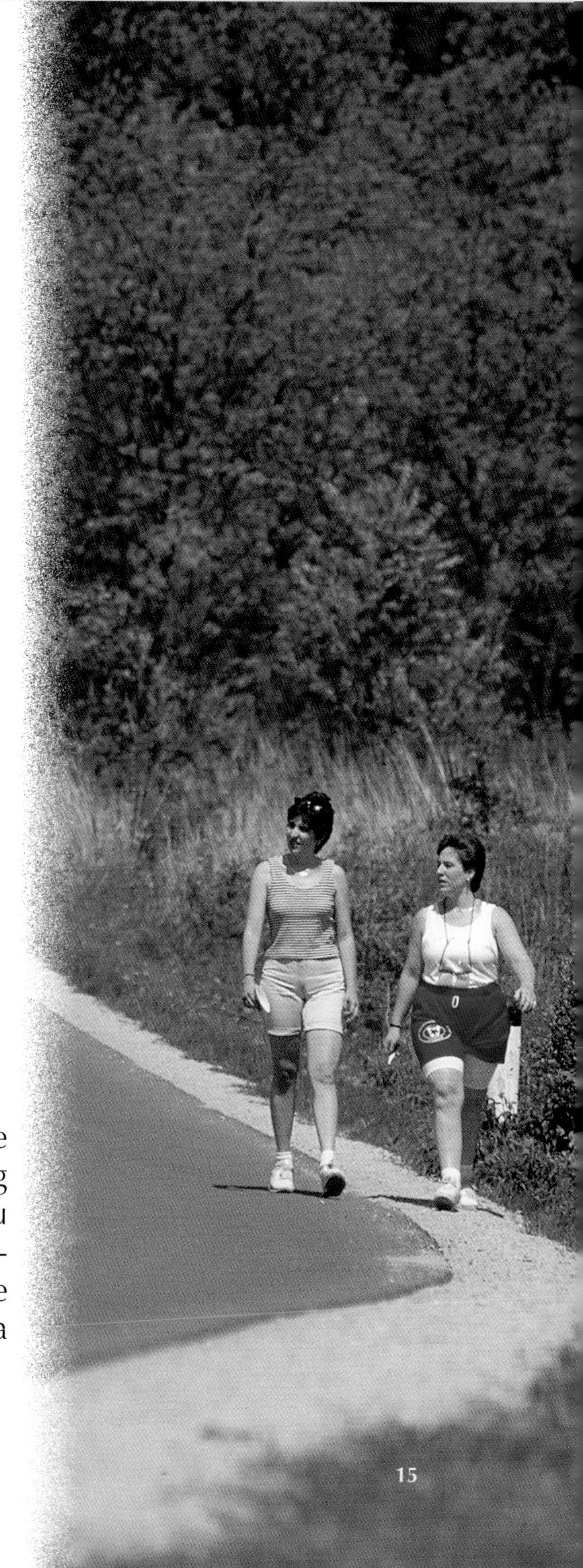

In This Chapter

- Taking a two-minute walk
- Turning downtime into opportunities for activity
- Turning light activity into moderate-intensity activity
- Checking out the benefits of walking
- Coming up with an activity plan

Now that you've completed your Personal Time Study, you know how much time you spend being active and inactive. This week we'll help you identify opportunities to turn some of those minutes of inactivity into activity. You'll discover the joys of a two-minute walk, and you'll draw up a plan for adding short walks to your schedule.

ACTIVITY ALERT

Let's Take a Walk!

We're going to begin by doing something not many authors do: We're going to ask you to stop reading. Why? We want you to take a walk.

Don't take a long hike, just a short, two-minute walk. Go up and down the corridor a few times, around the block, across the room and back several times—wherever you happen to be. Use a watch or clock to time yourself, and don't overdo it on your first time out. Walk, don't run, and for just two minutes—no more. When you're done, come back to this book and we'll compare notes.

Now take a walk.

Starting Off on the Right Foot

How did that feel? Did the two minutes go by quickly? If it's been a while since you've been active, you may have felt a little winded by the end of the walk. Did you want to stop? If you can make yourself walk for 2 minutes, over time you may find that 2 minutes can become 5 minutes, and eventually 5 minutes can become 10 minutes. If you can work up to at least three 10-minute brisk walks each day, you'll improve your fitness and get most other benefits of physical activity.

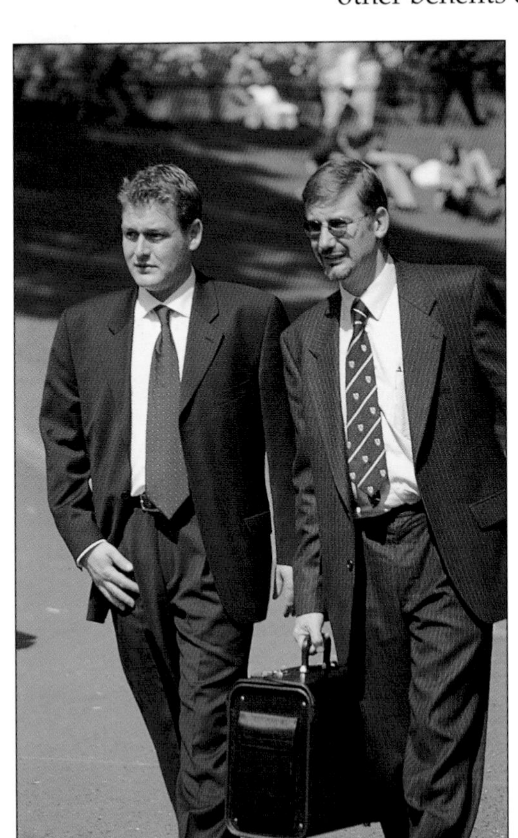

When and where can you take your two-minute walks?

Of course, the more you do, the better, but the official word from public health experts is that you should get at least 30 minutes of moderate-intensity physical activity on most, preferably all, days of the week.

First, let's concentrate on two-minute walks. One reason many people say they don't get enough exercise is that they don't have time, but everyone's got two minutes to spare now and then. The two-minute walk is an easy way to build activity into your day without taking a lot of time. You can do it almost anywhere and anytime. Here are a few suggestions:

- Get off the bus one block early and walk the rest of the way to work.
- Walk a block or two for lunch instead of going to the deli right across the street.
- Walk around for two minutes during your coffee break.
- Take a two-minute walk during TV commercials.

There's nothing inherently bad about watching TV, reading, or surfing the Internet. The problem is that most of us spend too much time in sedentary activities and not enough time moving. No, we're not going to ask you to give up something you love doing, but we are going to help you find time for more physical activity than you have been doing.

ACTIVITY ALERT

Turning Downtime Into Uptime

For starters, look at your Personal Time Study form on pages 11-12. Using the following form, make a list of each sedentary activity that filled your weekday. Then estimate how much time you spent doing each one.

Sedentary activity	Minutes a day
1.______________________	__________
2.______________________	__________
3.______________________	__________
4.______________________	__________
5.______________________	__________
6.______________________	__________

If you're surprised by how much time you spent sitting or stretched out on the sofa, don't despair. Now's the time to change that. Look back at your list and circle one sedentary activity that you can do less of. Logging 90 minutes a day in front of the tube? Maybe you can shorten that time by getting up and doing something during the commercial breaks. Surprised by how much time you spend on the telephone at home? Maybe you can walk while you talk using your portable phone. Write down your ideas for replacing sedentary activities with more active ones.

1.______________________

2.______________________

3.______________________

4.______________________

5.______________________

6.______________________

EXPERT ADVICE

Turning Light Activity Into Moderate Activity

You can also increase your daily physical activity by cranking up the intensity of light activities you already do each day. Moderate-intensity walking means walking a mile (1.6 km) in 15 to 20 minutes, a pace of three to four miles (4.8-6.4 km) an hour. It's roughly the way you walk when you're hurrying to make an appointment or to get out of the cold. Light-intensity activity is any physical activity more strenuous than sleeping and less strenuous than a brisk walk.

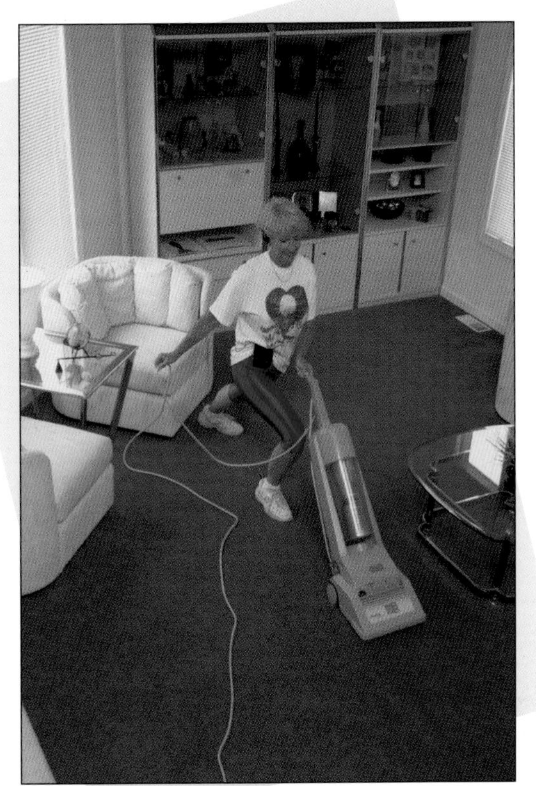

How can you add intensity to your light activities?

Here are a few clever ways our participants turned light activity into moderate-intensity activity:

- Let's say you usually stroll to the cafeteria on your afternoon break. Instead of lolling, take a brisk walk. You'll turn a light activity into a moderate one. (Go the long way around and you'll use even more energy.)
- When it's time to do some vacuuming at home, put on your favorite fast dance music and try to keep up. If you feel yourself getting slightly winded, then you're doing moderate-intensity activity.
- Love to shop? First take a fast-paced walk around the mall or shopping area, glancing at what the windows have to offer. Once you've completed your circuit, reward yourself by going back to check out things that intrigued you.

ACTIVITY ALERT

Planning for Moderate-Intensity Activities

Think about your daily schedule. What are some light activities you do that you could turn into moderate-intensity activities simply by picking up the pace? In the following space write down two light activities that you are willing to change.

Light-intensity activity	How I'll increase it to moderate-intensity activity
1. ____________	______________________________
2. ____________	______________________________

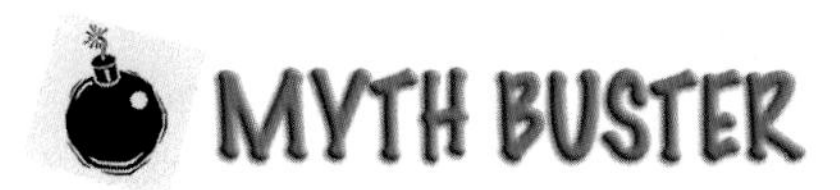

MYTH BUSTER

"I'm just too tired to walk now."

Studies show that being active makes people feel energetic. There are probably many reasons. For one thing, moving around helps get the blood flowing so you feel alert. Many people say they feel better about themselves when they are regularly active than when they are sedentary—more in control, more capable, more motivated. Plus, moderate exercise increases heart rate and breathing, which can improve overall fitness. The more fit you are, the more stamina you have for physical activity.

Why? As you become fit, your body improves its ability to use oxygen. Your heart improves its ability to supply blood to all parts of the body.

In fact, one thing you're likely to notice as you become fit is that your heart rate slows down. That's because it takes less effort to pump the same amount of blood to your brain and muscles than when you were unfit. A strong heart and cardiovascular system mean greater stamina and a decreased chance of heart attack.

Walking Works Wonders

By now, dozens of studies have confirmed the many health benefits associated with walking. Consider a few payoffs:

Weight control—The people who successfully lose weight, and keep it off, are people who incorporate physical activity into their weight-management plan. Even moderate-intensity activities such as brisk walking boost the calories you burn every day.

Good health—Many studies show that walking every day significantly reduces high blood pressure. Surprisingly, in fact, moderate-intensity activity seems to lower blood pressure better than vigorous exercise.

Bright spirits—Getting up and walking can help fight the blues. Some studies have shown that regular physical activity can help relieve stress and symptoms of depression.

High odds of staying healthy—People who make moderate activities such as walking part of everyday life run less risk of developing heart disease, colon cancer, and other chronic illnesses.

ACTIVITY ALERT

Coming Up With a Plan

You've given the two-minute walk a try, and you've found opportunities during the day when you can get up from your desk or sofa and get moving.

It's time to commit yourself to a plan. Identify where you can fit in a few two-minute walks this week. Maybe it's during your coffee break at work, or during commercials for your favorite TV show. Maybe you can park the car at the far

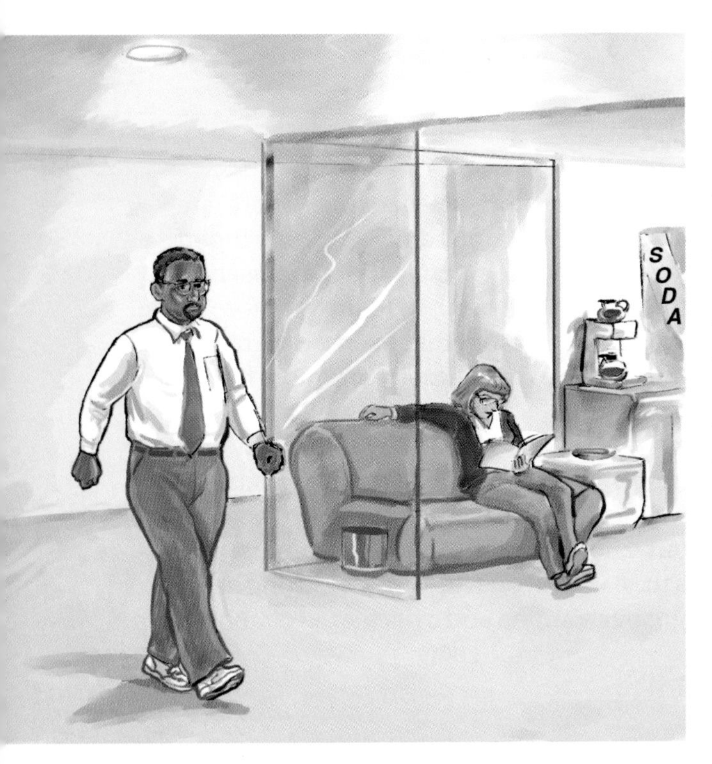

end of the lot or get off the bus a stop early and walk the rest of the way. If you're a new mom, you can strap on a Snuggly and take a refreshing walk. The point is to add a little more physical activity than what you have been accustomed to doing.

Use the following weekly calendar to identify when you will fit in at least one two-minute walk. (If you can do more, that's great.) Be specific. Our research shows that the more specific your plan, the more likely you are to follow it. For example, you might decide to do a two-minute walk Monday, Wednesday, and Friday during your lunch hour, or perhaps you'll decide to walk during the commercial breaks following the news.

Use your breaks at work to take a two-minute walk.

MY PLAN FOR TWO-MINUTE WALKS

Monday

Tuesday

Wednesday

Thursday

Friday

Saturday

Sunday

DID YOU KNOW?

The total number of calories you expend is the same whether you do three 10-minute bouts of activity or one 30-minute session (as long as the intensity remains the same). If you're busy, chances are it's easier to find several opportunities for short activities than an uninterrupted half hour. If you're overweight or obese, it may be easier to accumulate shorter bouts during the day. A research group at the University of Pittsburgh[3] has shown that obese women found it easier to stick with a program of four 10-minute bouts of activity over time than one 40-minute bout. The group of obese women who added four 10-minute bouts ended up burning a greater number of calories and tended to lose more weight than the group of obese women who did one 40-minute bout per day.

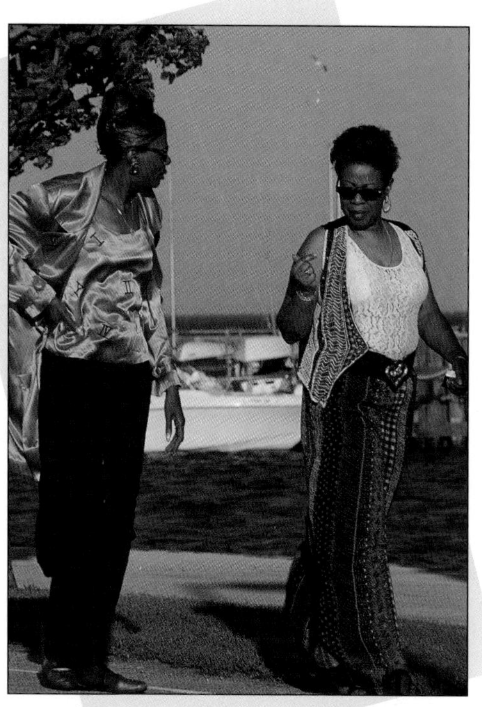

It may be easier to accumulate short bouts of exercise during the day than to walk a full 30 or more minutes at one time.

EXPERT ADVICE

Any time you try to make a big change in your life—whether you're adding activity, losing weight, or quitting smoking—it's easy to get discouraged. But don't let that sideline your efforts to change. Here are two simple tips to remember:

1. Lasting changes begin with small steps.

Once you've made up your mind to change, it's natural to want to jump right in and do it. There's nothing wrong with being gung ho. But too often, people who start with a big bang end up fizzling before the first lap is over. They buy that gym membership, plunge into a new routine, and the next day they're so sore and tired they have to take the rest of the week off. Right away they feel discouraged, and soon the gym shoes begin gathering dust in the closet.

The best way to make a *lasting* change is to begin gradually, reward yourself along the way, and plan for times when you fall behind.

2. Doing something is better than doing nothing.

The latest findings—some of it from our own research—show that adding short stretches of activity during the day can make a difference. You don't have to do your exercise all at once. Doing 10 minutes of moderate-intensity activities three times a day can add up to big health benefits.

No matter how busy you are, you can find a few minutes. Ask most people why they don't get as much exercise as they know they should, and the answer is usually the same: no time. It's easy to understand. With clamoring kids and long commutes, errands to run and people to see, most of us don't have enough time for everything we'd like to do. There's even less time for the things we know we *should* do. That's the most important lesson of the two-minute walk. Most commercial breaks on television run longer than two minutes. With all the stations on cable TV these days, it takes longer than that to click through to see what's on. Two minutes is about as long as it takes to heat up water for tea in the microwave. No matter how busy you are, chances are you have two-minute stretches of time here and there.

UP CLOSE & PERSONAL

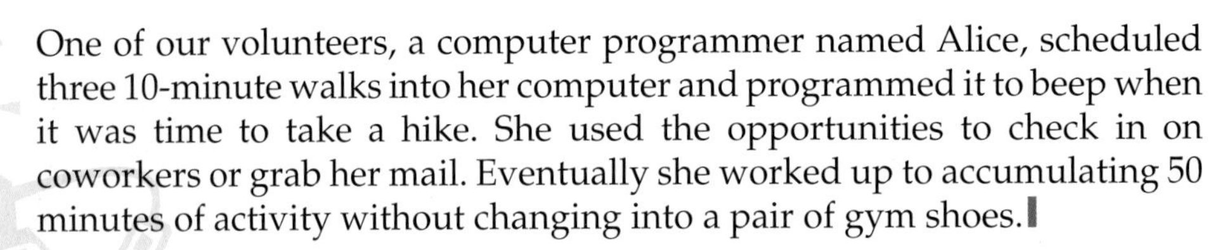

One of our volunteers, a computer programmer named Alice, scheduled three 10-minute walks into her computer and programmed it to beep when it was time to take a hike. She used the opportunities to check in on coworkers or grab her mail. Eventually she worked up to accumulating 50 minutes of activity without changing into a pair of gym shoes.

Chapter Checklist

Before you move on to the next week's activities, make sure you

- Identified inactive periods during the day that you can turn into activity
- Found at least three ways to turn light activity into moderate-intensity activity
- Made a plan for adding a few two-minute walks to your schedule this week

Once you've practiced the two-minute walk, it's time to look at some obstacles that can get in the way of achieving your goal. For most of us, there are plenty of hurdles to get over. The good news is that there are just as many clever ways to overcome those obstacles and become active.

WEEK **FOUR**

Barriers and Benefits

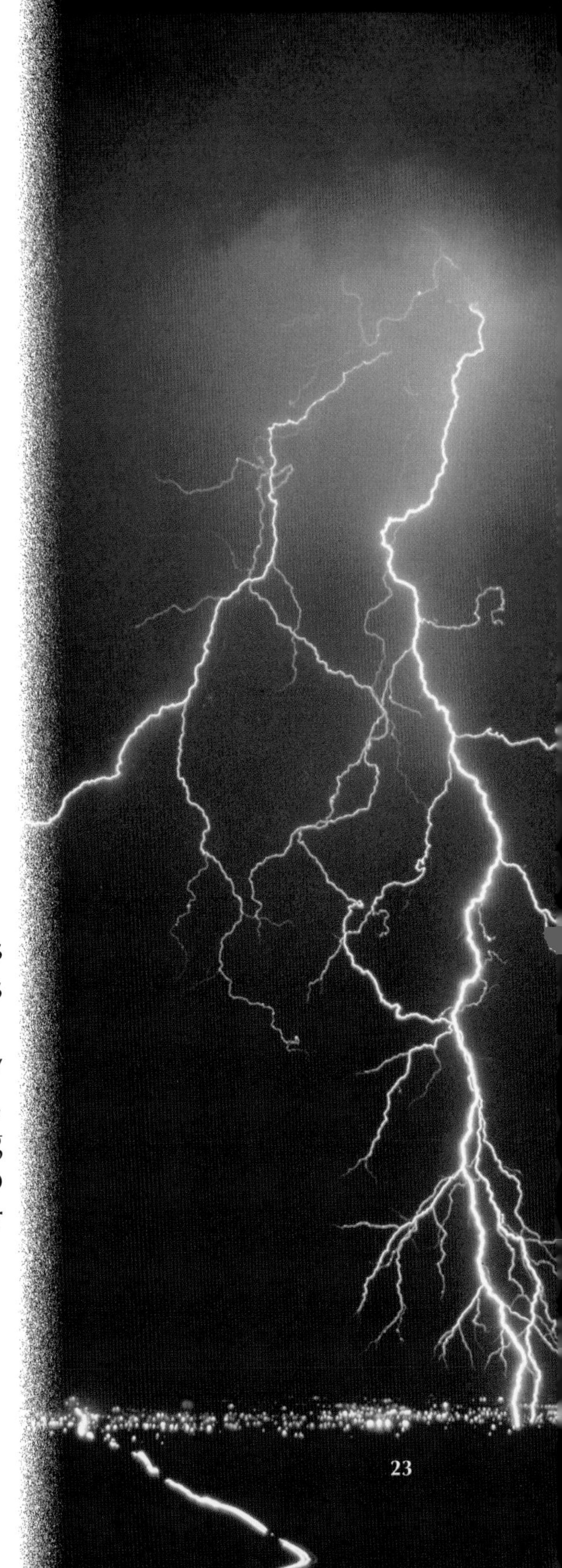

In This Chapter

- Looking beyond the usual excuses
- Identifying the barriers you face
- Reviewing the benefits of an active life

Health experts can point to plenty of good reasons most of us should increase our activity. Chances are you've got a few of your own.

You probably also have plenty of reasons why it's hard to follow through. You're busy at work, relatives are visiting, or the holidays are coming up. Your reasons may be valid, but they can also be barriers that keep you from achieving your goals.

This week, while you follow your plan for fitting two-minute walks into your daily schedule, we're going to look at the barriers that may be getting in your way. To overcome barriers, first we have to identify them. That's what this week is about.

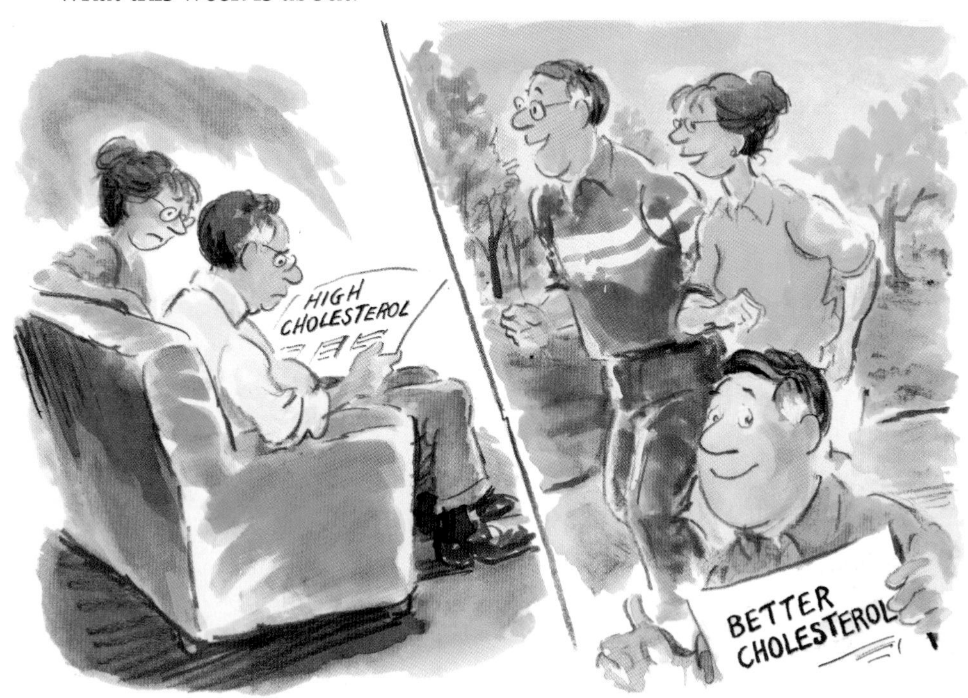

Excuses, Excuses

Why do the best-laid plans so often fall apart? Here are the three leading reasons we've heard from participants in our physical activity programs:

"I Just Don't Have the Time"

Nice try, but remember what we said in the last chapter: we all have the same number of hours—168 to be exact—at our disposal each week. What varies is what we choose to do with those hours. Everyone has some leisure time to spend reading, watching TV, daydreaming, e-mailing, or chatting on the telephone. The question is this: Which of these activities can you cut back on to fit in additional physical activity each day? Are you willing to substitute some physical activity for something else you spend your time on now?

"I Don't Know How to Exercise"

Some people are sedentary because they think they don't know how to exercise properly. Because they have never developed exercise skills, they may lack self-confidence. But you don't need any special skill to put one foot in front of another and enjoy a brisk walk. That's the whole point of adding simple, everyday activities to your life. You don't need special skills or fancy equipment.

"I Can't Get the Help I Need"

We all have people around us who influence what we do and what we don't do. Those people can have a big role to play when we're trying to make a change in our lives. Sometimes they can help. Unfortunately, sometimes they can hinder. If the people around you—your spouse, coworkers, or friends—*aren't* supportive, succeeding can be tough. Research has shown that having the support of friends and family members is especially important for adopting new physical activity habits. Later we'll show you some tips on how to get the support you need.

UP CLOSE & PERSONAL

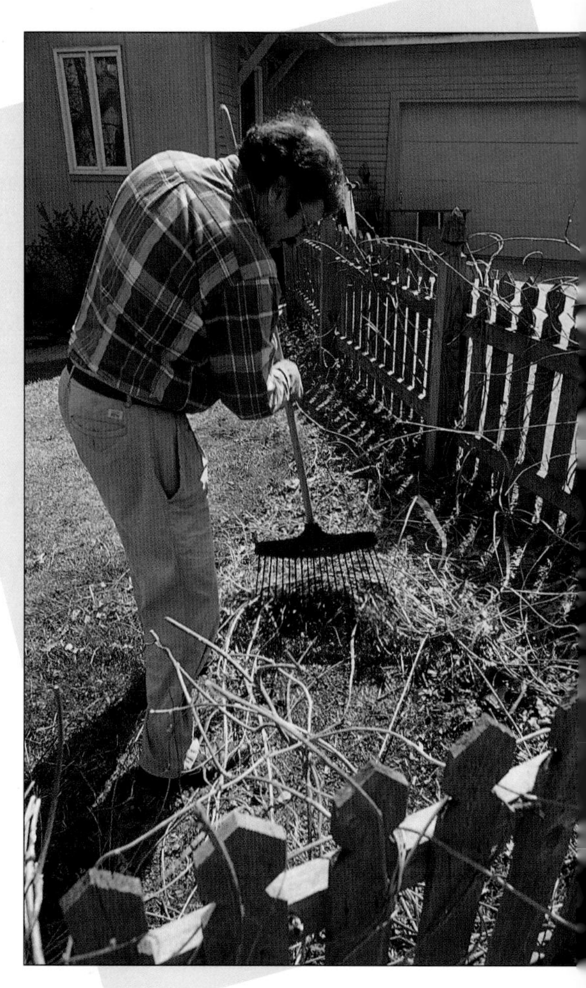

As a kid, George wasn't good at sports. Ever since, he's shied away from exercise.

Now in his 40s, George realizes how important becoming physically active is to his health. So he joined a club and started lifting weights and jogging. After the second day he was so sore he could hardly get out of bed. He figured he was too old to start getting into shape and quit altogether. The bad experience confirmed his sense that exercise wasn't for him.

George's downfall was a lack of knowledge about how to start increasing physical activity. He could have benefited from a few solid pieces of advice. First, choose activities you like to do. (George liked to garden and work in his yard, for instance.) Also, take it slowly. Even moderate-intensity activities such as gardening provide important health benefits. The most important goal is to turn activity into a lifetime habit.

Luckily, George didn't give up. In our program, he learned that there are many ways to be active and that doing what you love is the best way to become active and stick with it. These days, George works in his garden every chance he gets. He has never felt better in his life, and his garden has never looked more beautiful.

MYTH BUSTER

"You can't tell me gardening counts as exercise."

Sure we can. Raking leaves, mowing the grass with a push mower, or digging a new flower or vegetable bed all count as moderate- to vigorous-intensity activities, depending on how hard you go at them. (Sitting on your haunches and pulling weeds or planting seeds doesn't count.)

Working Through Barriers

For the participants in our program, lack of time was one of the most common barriers, but every person has his or her own personal barriers. For example, one woman had lots of time but had to care for her elderly mother, which left her too tired to do activities for herself. One man in our study had never thought of himself as an active person, although he liked to follow sports and had a library of books about legendary athletes.

Each of these people found themselves facing tall hurdles, but not insurmountable ones. The woman taking care of her mother arranged for other family members to provide care for two afternoons a week. She fit in physical activity on those days and early in the morning before her mother woke up. The increased activity soon helped her feel less tired.

The man who loved to follow sports but was rarely active himself realized that you don't have to be a serious athlete to be active. He had always loved going to the local playing field on Saturdays to watch softball games. He began going half an hour early and walking briskly around the field before the game. During breaks in the action he took a lap or two around the field. It didn't take long before he began to think of himself as an active person.

ACTIVITY ALERT

Identifying My Physical Activity Barriers

Now we want you to identify your physical activity barriers. As you go through the week, be conscious of anything that seems to get in the way of your plan, and add it to the list.

1. ____________________

2. ____________________

3. ____________________

4. ____________________

5. ____________________

6. ____________________

7. ____________________

8. ____________________

ACTIVITY ALERT

Identifying Benefits of Physical Activity

One way to motivate yourself to get over barriers is to remember the important benefits physical activity can provide. All of us have one or two things that are especially important—benefits that are powerful enough to get us going even when we're not in the mood. Benefits our participants listed include: feeling productive, enjoying improved communication with a spouse, and feeling good about their bodies. It's important to identify the benefits that matter to *you*. Take a few minutes now to list the most important benefits you can gain by exercising. Again, as you go through your week, keep adding to your list.

1. ______________________________
2. ______________________________
3. ______________________________
4. ______________________________
5. ______________________________
6. ______________________________
7. ______________________________
8. ______________________________

EXPERT ADVICE

Now for an Encouraging Word

The evidence from scientific studies is as solid as a rock: Physical activity is crucial to good health and overall well-being. Here's what we know for certain.

- People who are physically active are less likely than people who are inactive to die of heart disease and some types of cancer, such as colon cancer.
- As they get older, active people have a better quality of life and suffer fewer disabilities than inactive people.
- Physical activity helps keep blood pressure down, minimizes bone loss

as we age, and lowers the risk of developing non-insulin dependent diabetes.

- Physical activity helps people maintain their weight effectively.
- People who are regularly active report feeling less stressed and more able to cope with life than when they were inactive. They are less likely to feel depressed or anxious than sedentary people.
- Many people in physical activity studies report feeling more energetic and productive than before they increased their activity.
- People who become physically active often report sleeping better than when they were inactive.

? DID YOU KNOW?

Moderate-intensity exercise could help you ward off cold and flu bugs. Not long ago, exercise physiologist David Nieman and colleagues[4] followed 32 women—some of whom got no exercise and some of whom took up walking. After 12 weeks, the nonwalkers reported twice as many days with cold or flu symptoms as the walkers. Blood tests showed that the women in the walking group had boosted their immune systems. Since then, many other studies have shown that moderate exercise—a 30-minute brisk walk most days of the week—can bolster the body's immune defenses.

By now you've given some thought to the reasons you aren't as active as you'd like to be. Confronting the obstacles you face is the first step in overcoming them. Sometimes barriers can seem overwhelming. If you feel that way about becoming physically active, remind yourself of the benefits of being active. Long-term benefits such as lower risk of heart disease and other chronic illnesses are important, of course. If these seem too far away to offer much motivation, however, remember that there are also quick rewards to getting up and moving, such as an improved outlook or increased energy.

Chapter Checklist

Before you move on to the next week's activities, make sure you

- [ ] Identified at least three barriers that prevent you from being active
- [ ] Listed at least three important benefits of increasing your activity

In this week you've had a chance to discover the barriers you face. In the next week we'll look at successful strategies for overcoming your barriers.

WEEK **FIVE**

Over, Under, Around, and Through

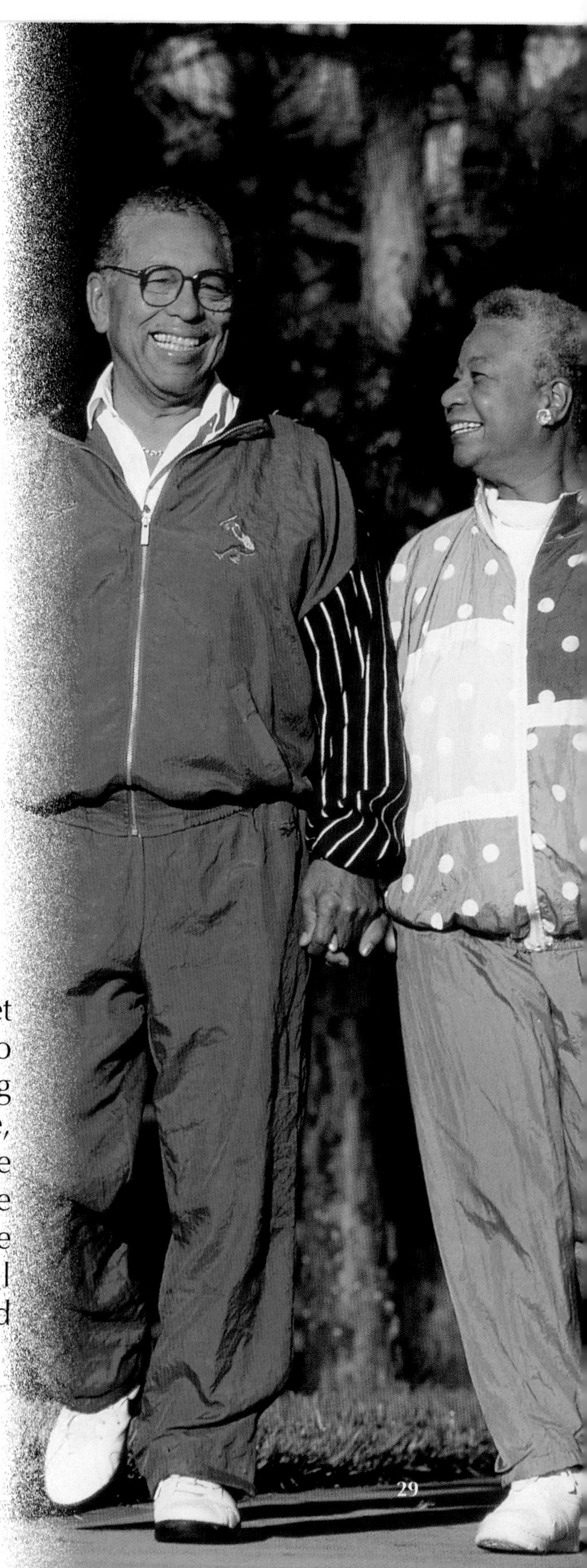

In This Chapter

- Learning the art of problem solving
- Coming up with ways to get around barriers
- Looking back at stages of change

By now you've made a list of the barriers that get in the way of your physical activity. You've also listed the benefits you'd like to get by increasing your activity. If you're like most inactive people, your list of barriers is longer than benefits. Take heart. There are plenty of ways around those barriers. The more active you become, the more important the benefits will be. This week, we'll develop strategies for getting over, under, and around barriers.

EXPERT ADVICE

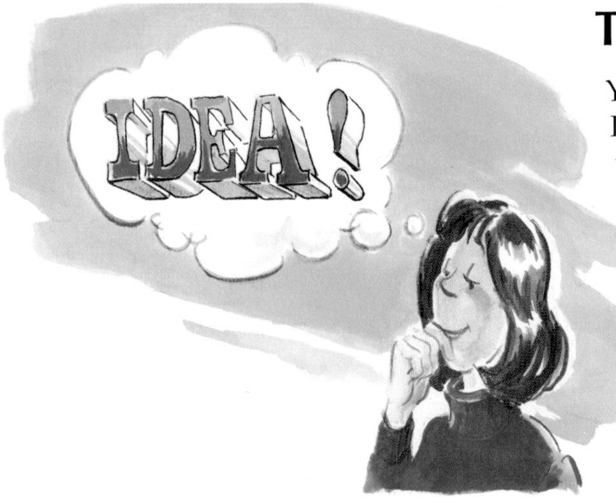

The Art of Problem Solving

You've already taken the most important step: Identifying your personal barriers. The next step is to use some simple problem-solving skills. There's nothing fancy about it. Problem solving simply means thinking creatively about the most effective solution to use when a problem—or an obstacle—blocks your way. Behavioral scientists have devised many problem-solving models. Here's a simple approach that seemed to work well for participants in our program. Just think IDEA.

ACTIVITY ALERT

Think IDEA

Identify the Problem

You've already done most of the work here. From the list you made in week 4, select one barrier. Write it down on the "Good Idea!" form on the next page. Take a moment to think about the specifics. What in particular about this barrier keeps you from being active? Perhaps you are having trouble being active on your many business trips. Travel may make you feel too tired to be physically active, or perhaps you don't feel safe or comfortable walking or doing other activities in an unfamiliar place. Maybe you just don't have time. Chances are it's a combination of factors. Write down the most important specifics about your personal barrier so you don't forget.

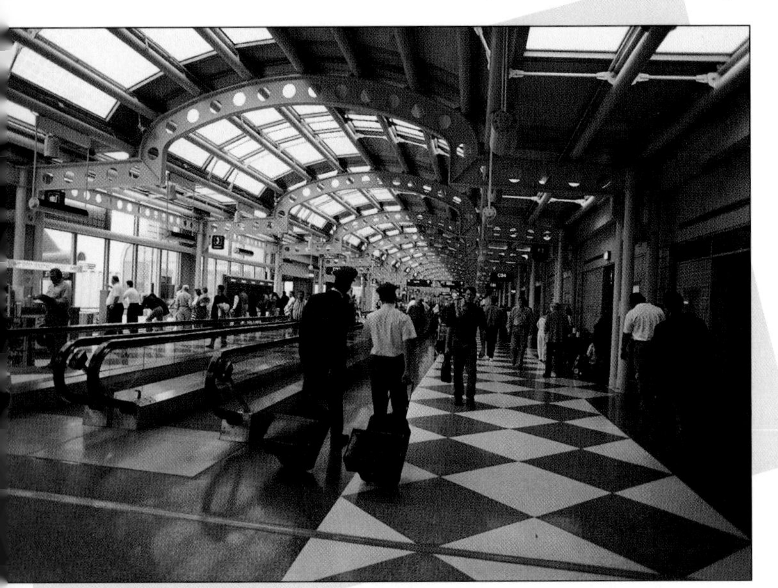
Even if you travel a lot, you can find ways to be active at the airport or the hotel.

Develop a List of Solutions

That means brainstorming—getting down to business and coming up with ideas. Be creative. Don't worry whether the solutions are good or bad, workable or unrealistic. That will come later. Sometimes your wildest idea will turn out to be the best solution. Jot down all the ideas you can come up with. Keep your list with you over the next few days and add any other solutions that come to mind.

Evaluate Your Solutions

Some will look more realistic than others. One that seemed far-fetched may begin to look interesting. Select one that you're willing to try, then develop a specific plan for how and when you can put it to the test. Here's what a plan might look like. Let's say your downfall is business trips, and the problem is that you don't feel comfortable walking in an unfamiliar area. One plan might involve checking ahead to make sure your hotel has an exercise facility. Another plan might involve learning a set of simple aerobics exercises you can take on the road and do in the comfort and privacy of your hotel room. A third strategy might be walking as much as you can instead of sitting at the airport.

Analyze How Well Your Plan Worked

After you have given your plan a try, analyze how well it worked. Be honest. This is the time to revise your plan before you try again. Maybe all you need is a little tinkering, but if the plan fell flat on its face, come up with another by starting at the beginning of the IDEA process.

GREAT IDEA!

I—Identify a barrier that keeps you from being active.

____

____

____

D—Develop a few creative solutions (the more the merrier).

____

____

____

E—Evaluate your list of solutions. In the following space, write the solution you are willing to try. While you're at it, write down precisely *when* you will put it into action.

____

____

____

A—Analyze how well your plan worked and revise it if necessary. If your plan worked well, give it five stars. If it only deserves two stars, write down how it could become a five-star plan. If your plan bombed completely, look back at your list of solutions and try again. (Remember, a plan that doesn't work isn't a complete failure. It often points toward the solution that *will* work. The only failure is giving up.)

____

____

____

Use the "Great IDEA!" form whenever you find a problem you need to solve. You may photocopy the form in this book for your own use.

UP CLOSE & PERSONAL

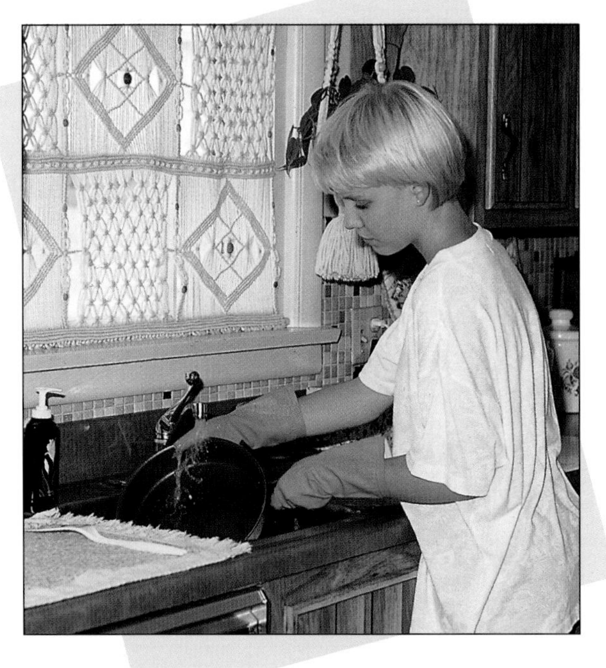

Ida had plenty of reasons to increase her activity, including losing a few unwanted pounds. With three teenagers at home and a job as an office manager for a large construction company, however, she never seemed to find the time.

Ida decided to identify the barriers that kept her from being active. First there was the rush to get the kids and herself out the door so she could be at her desk at 7 A.M. Though she was allowed a 15-minute break in the morning, she usually didn't take it. Even during her half-hour lunch break, she typically ate a sandwich at her desk. She got off work at 3:30—just in time to pick up her youngest, run errands, do a little housework, or go watch the other kids play baseball. In the evening, while the kids did homework, she usually ironed, fixed lunch, and sometimes watched a little TV. By 9:30 she was ready for bed. Thinking about it made her realize what a treadmill she was on—just not the right one.

So over lunch one day, Ida began developing solutions. Within 20 minutes she had about 20 ideas—some reasonable, some zany. Here's part of her list:

- Aerobic telephoning while ordering building materials
- Taking a 10-minute walk at lunch and break time
- Walking around the baseball field during the kids' games
- Walking to the corner grocery store instead of driving
- Taking a talk-and-walk with her husband two nights a week instead of watching their usual game show
- Asking the kids to take over a few household chores (with a little extra allowance thrown in) to give her a time for a brisk walk through the neighborhood after dinner

After evaluating all her ideas, Ida chose one; she decided to ask her husband to walk for half an hour instead of sitting in front of television. They agreed to think of it as a date. Ida was surprised to discover how wonderful the time spent together was. They talked about the kids, their work, the neighborhood. Before long they went from two nights a week to three.

A few weeks later, Ida took a few minutes to analyze how well her solution was working. In fact, she was delighted with her progress—so delighted that she went back to her list of solutions and selected another: walking around the baseball field during the kids' games.

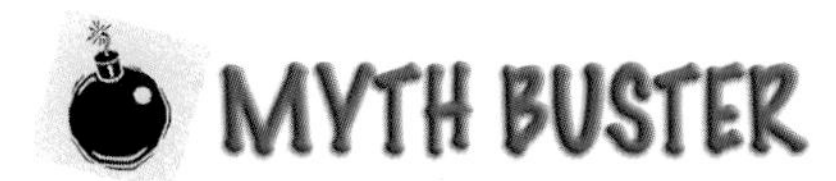

A lifetime of physical activity may protect against several forms of cancer. Scientists at the Harvard School of Public Health in Boston found that men who remained physically active throughout their lives were half as likely as their sedentary counterparts to develop colon cancer.[5] Other studies suggest that exercise may lower the risk of prostate cancer and breast cancer.

MYTH BUSTER

"I've tried and failed so many times, I'm beginning to think I'm not cut out for exercise."

Overcoming Myths

- Slips can help us see how to change our plans.
- *Every*body's body was designed to be physically active—even yours!

There are two myths at work here. First is the idea that slipping now and then means you've failed. The truth is, no one succeeds without a few slips along the way. Slips can even point the way by spotlighting obstacles or showing where your plan needs tinkering. The second myth is that some people aren't cut out for exercise. Exercise is just a fancy word for physical activity, after all. Let's face it: Our bodies were designed to be physically active. That doesn't mean all of us have to like going to an aerobics class, but all of us have some kinds of physical activity we can enjoy and feel good at.

ACTIVITY ALERT

How Are You Doing?

Now that the first few weeks are almost done, it's time for a progress report. Chances are you've had some new insights about how you spend your time, and you've come up with some great ideas to turn sedentary time into active time. You may even find yourself in a different stage on your way to making lasting change. The questions in the flow chart should be familiar: You answered them in week 2. Take a few minutes to look at them again. Be honest. If you've taken a step forward in the stages of change, congratulations! If not, don't fret. We're not giving out awards here. Even if you're only thinking about activity more than you were, that's moving in the right direction.

What stage are you in now? Have you made progress? Now's the time to look again at the references in appendix B that contain advice for each stage of change. If you're in the action stage (doing the new habit consistently but for less than six months), take a look at "Sticking to It" on page 176, where you'll find a list of benefits to help keep you motivated. If you're in the stage of contemplation (giving it a thought now and then, but not doing it), read "Try It, You'll Like It" on page 175, which contains helpful hints to move you on to preparation.

Health experts now know that being inactive is a problem for many people—a big problem that can rob them of health, energy, and even happiness. Luckily, like most problems, you can solve inactivity with a little ingenuity and persistence. This week, you've identified one of your biggest

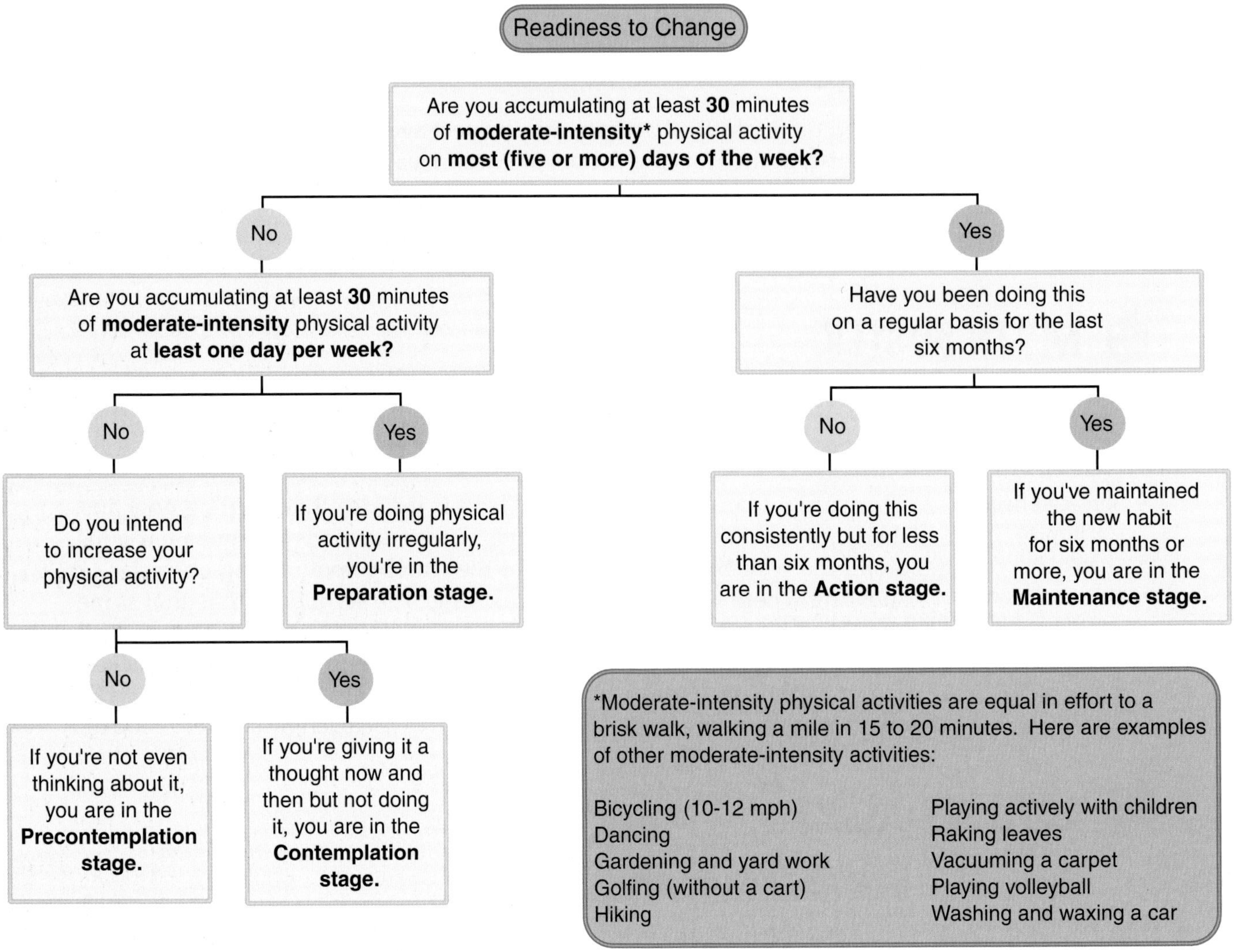

Readiness to Change

Are you accumulating at least **30** minutes of **moderate-intensity*** physical activity on **most (five or more) days of the week?**

- **No** → Are you accumulating at least **30** minutes of **moderate-intensity** physical activity at **least one day per week?**
  - **No** → Do you intend to increase your physical activity?
    - **No** → If you're not even thinking about it, you are in the **Precontemplation stage.**
    - **Yes** → If you're giving it a thought now and then but not doing it, you are in the **Contemplation stage.**
  - **Yes** → If you're doing physical activity irregularly, you're in the **Preparation stage.**
- **Yes** → Have you been doing this on a regular basis for the last six months?
  - **No** → If you're doing this consistently but for less than six months, you are in the **Action stage.**
  - **Yes** → If you've maintained the new habit for six months or more, you are in the **Maintenance stage.**

*Moderate-intensity physical activities are equal in effort to a brisk walk, walking a mile in 15 to 20 minutes. Here are examples of other moderate-intensity activities:

Bicycling (10-12 mph)
Dancing
Gardening and yard work
Golfing (without a cart)
Hiking
Playing actively with children
Raking leaves
Vacuuming a carpet
Playing volleyball
Washing and waxing a car

obstacles and developed some solutions. You've also evaluated those solutions, then analyzed what works and what doesn't for you. No matter what problems you face, these steps offer a useful way to understand what you're up against and find ways around it.

If you're stuck in a rut, look back at the last two weeks to find ways to encourage and motivate yourself.

Chapter Checklist

Before you move on to the next week's activities, make sure you

- ☐ Filled out the Great IDEA! form
- ☐ Revisited the Readiness to Change form to chart your progress

In the next week, we're going to ask you to get ready to do a little math. We'll also show you a nifty way to tally up your energy expenditure: how many calories you burn doing different physical activities.

WEEK SIX

Let's Burn Some Calories!

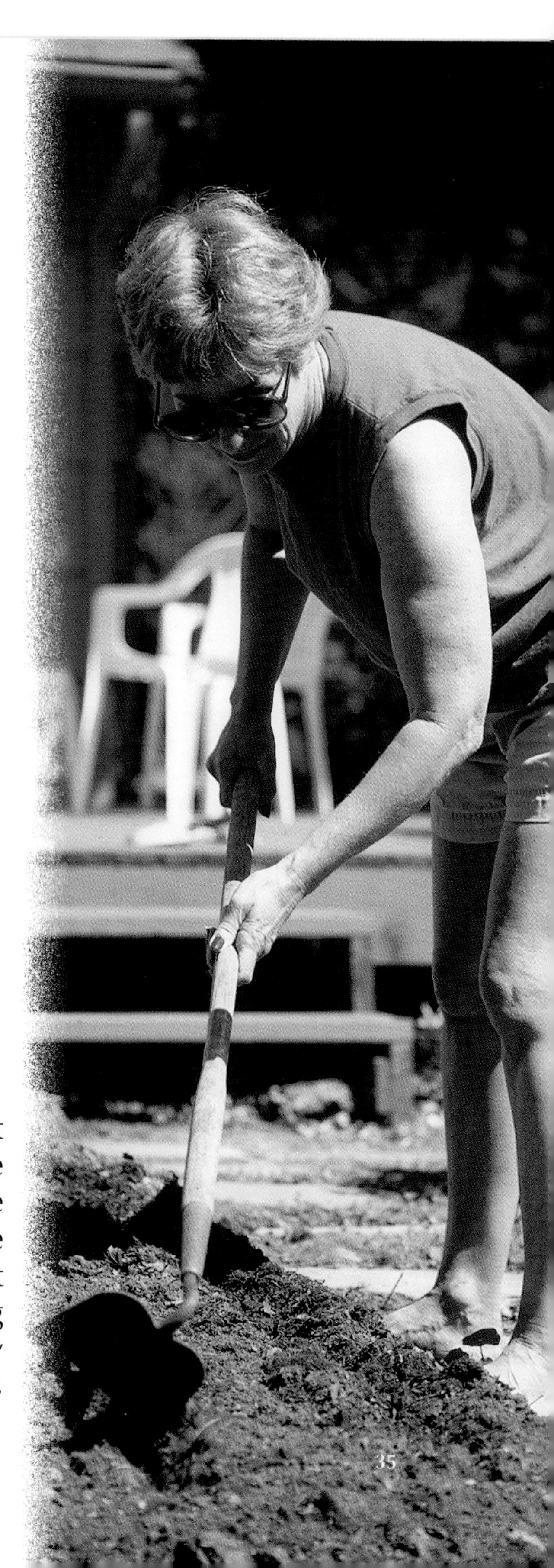

In This Chapter

- Recognizing factors that impact physical activity energy expenditure
- Identifying light-, moderate-, and vigorous-intensity activities
- Calculating ways to burn an extra 1,000 calories per week
- Completing simple fitness tests

To reach a goal, you need to start with a plan. Just as important, you have to know how to measure your progress. So far you've been adding up the amount of time you spend every day doing some kind of physical activity. This week, we'll look at another way of measuring progress—calculating how much energy you burn being physically active. Why is this important? Research shows

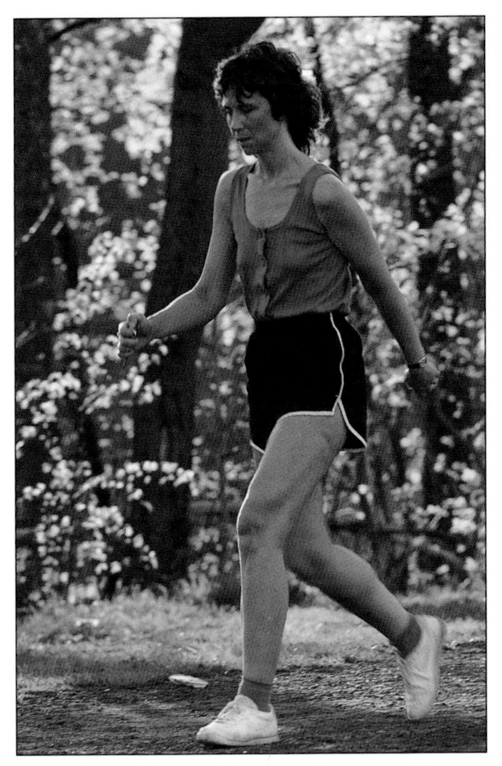

Regardless of the activity you choose and how often you do it, what matters is how much energy you expend over a day, week, or month.

that regardless of whether you do your activity in short bouts or long bouts, at a moderate intensity or a vigorous intensity, what matters is how much energy you expend over a day, week, or month. In fact, the U.S. Surgeon General recommends burning at least 1,000 calories a week in physical activities. Remember these numbers. We'll come back to them later.

Energy expenditure depends on four simple things:

- your current body weight, how hard you push yourself (intensity),
- the amount of time you engage in an activity (duration), and
- how often you do the activity (frequency).

Together, body size, intensity, duration, and frequency can tell you roughly how many calories you are burning while you're physically active. Let's examine this closely.

EXPERT ADVICE

Body Size Does Matter

A 200-pound (90.7 kg) person is going to burn more calories than a 140-pound (63.5 kg) person doing the same activity. Why? The larger body has more mass to move around. Try this experiment. Take a walk around the block or up a couple flights of stairs. Then load yourself down with 10 to 20 extra pounds (4.5-9.1 kg). Put some bricks or canned goods in a bag or day pack. Walk around the block a second time. How did it feel? We'll bet you were working harder (i.e., burning more calories) than your first trip. Compare Flora who weights only 140 pounds with Tom who tips the scale at 200 pounds:

	Estimated calories burned per minute	
	Flora 140 lb (63.5 kg)	**Tom 200 lb (90.7 kg)**
Walking at moderate pace 20 min. per mile (1.6 km)	3.7	5.3

It is easy to see from this table that, walking at the same speed, Tom burns more calories per minute than Flora. His heart, lungs, and muscles are working harder than Flora's to move his bigger body. Therefore, he burns more calories.

A Close Look at Intensity

Next, let's look at exercise intensity. You probably realize that for a given time, the more vigorous the activity, the more energy (calories) you burn. Again, compare Flora and Tom as they do different activities.

	Estimated calories burned per minute		
Physical activity	**Intensity category**	**Flora 140 lb (63.5 kg)**	**Tom 200 lb (90.7 kg)**
Walking			
30 min. per mile (1.6 km) pace	Light	2.8	4.0
20 min. per mile	Moderate	3.7	5.3
15 min. per mile	Moderate	5.6	8.0
12 min. per mile	Very hard	9.0	12.7
Mowing lawn			
Riding mower	Light	2.8	4.0
Power mower, walk behind	Moderate	5.0	7.2
Hand mower, no power	Hard	6.7	9.6

This table shows how two common activities, walking and lawn mowing, can burn different numbers of calories depending on the intensity of the activity. Once again, you can see how different Flora's and Tom's energy expenditures are for each intensity level because of their body weight.

For comparison, let's think of intensity ranging from light and medium to hard and very hard. Exercise physiologists classify *light* activities as those that burn 1 to 3 times the energy as the body at complete rest. *Moderate* activities are those that burn 3 to 5 times the energy as the body at rest. *Hard* and *very hard* activities burn 5 to 7 and 7 or more times the energy as the body at rest, respectively. Let's look at where some common activities fall in terms of intensity.

Light

Working at a desk, standing, cooking, chopping vegetables, driving a car, light cleaning, watching TV, and reading.

Moderate

Brisk walking, raking, weeding, mopping, sweeping, light weightlifting, doing calisthenics, golfing (no cart), biking at a slow pace (around 10 miles [16 km] an hour), or paddling in a pool.

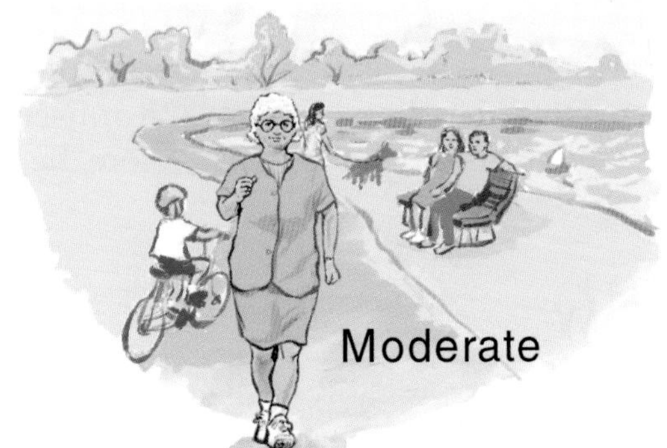
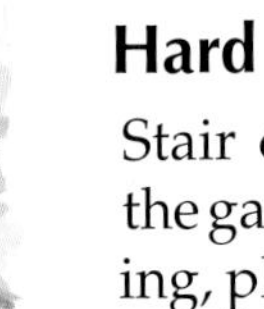

Hard

Stair climbing, scrubbing the floor, digging in the garden, doing heavy carpentry, aerobic dancing, playing doubles tennis, biking at a medium pace (around 13 miles [20.9 km] an hour), or swimming laps.

Very Hard

Chopping wood, carrying heavy loads, playing singles tennis, playing soccer or basketball, jumping rope, running, biking at a fast pace (more than 14 miles [22.5 km] an hour), or doing hard physical labor such as digging a ditch or hauling rocks.

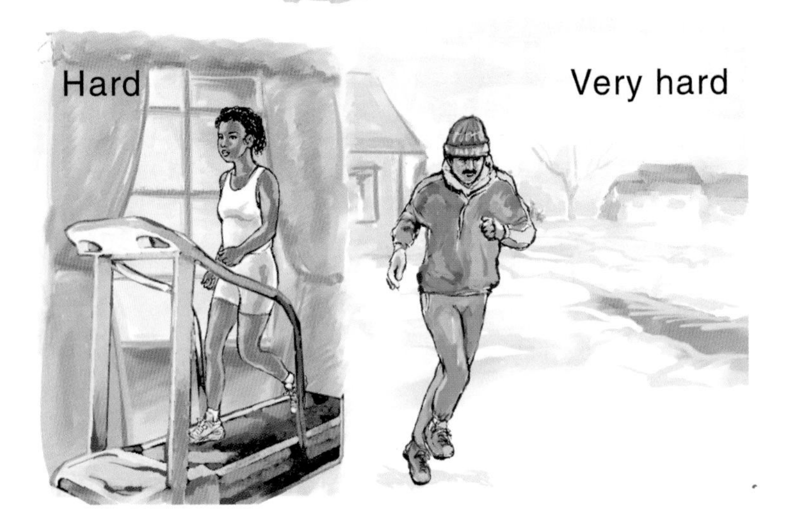

ACTIVITY ALERT

Checking Your Pace

One good way to understand intensity is to pay attention to how physical activity feels as you're doing it. Try a simple experiment. Map out a one-half mile (.8 km) course in your neighborhood. A good place to start is the local high school. Many have one-quarter mile (.4 km) tracks. One day this week, walk the course at your usual pace for one-half mile (.8 km), keeping track of your time. Record your time on this page. Then use the time to determine the approximate intensity of your activity:

My time for the one-half mile (.8 km) circuit is ________.

Now compare your time with the following chart. How are you doing?

Time	Intensity
More than 10 minutes	Light
7.5 to 10 minutes	Moderate
6 to 7.5 minutes	Hard intensity (chances are you're jogging)
Less than 6	Very hard intensity (we know you're running)

How Hard Do I Need to Push Myself?

There was a time, not long ago, when exercise gurus made a big deal about exercise intensity. To get the benefits of exercise, they said, you needed to reach your target heart rate, then stay there for a certain time, and that meant working up a serious sweat. OK, we'll admit it: we said the same thing ourselves. And we still think it's good advice for those who wish to engage in structured exercise and improve their fitness to a high level. However, what most Americans need is simply to increase their physical activity. The good news is that for most people, regularly doing moderate-intensity activities such as brisk walking, playing golf, or working in the yard offers important health benefits.

So the answer to the intensity question depends on who you are and what you want to achieve. Think for a moment about your starting position and your reasons for wanting to increase your activity. If you're sedentary or unfit, moderate-intensity activities will increase your fitness level and provide health benefits such as reduced blood pressure or cholesterol. If you're already active and in good shape, you may need to do hard or very hard activities to improve your fitness and further reduce your health risks.

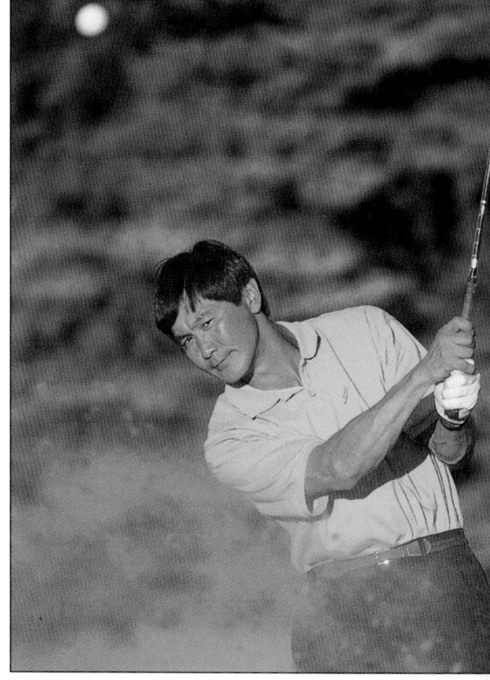

Even moderate-intensity activities like walking the golf course offer important health benefits.

In It for the Duration

We've shown that body weight and exercise intensity are important to overall energy expenditure. But so are the duration and frequency of your physical activity. Let's go back to Flora and Tom. As the following table shows, the longer you do an activity, the more calories you burn.

	Estimated calories burned					
	Flora 140 lb (63.5 kg)			Tom 200 lb (90.7 kg)		
	Minutes			Minutes		
	10	30	60	10	30	60
Walking						
30 min. per mile (1.6 km) pace	28	94	168	44	132	264
20 min. per mile	37	111	222	53	159	318
15 min. per mile	56	168	336	80	240	480
12 min. per mile	90	270	540	127	381	762

We have told you that you don't have to do all your physical activity in a 30-minute block of time. If you are going to be physically active only a couple days a week, you will need to remain active for longer periods each time than if you were active five days a week. If you can be active every day, you can build in minisessions several times each day of the week. Do whatever works best for you.

We said earlier in the chapter that people should burn at least 1,000 extra calories a week. How can you do this? By increasing the intensity, duration, and frequency, the possibilities are endless! Here is how Flora planned to burn 1,000 extra calories one week.

Physical activity	Calories per minute*	Total time (minutes)	Total calories (calories per minute × total time)
Moderate			
Walking, 20 min. per mile (1.6 km)	3.7	120	444
Mowing lawn, power mower	5.0	30	150
Vacuuming vigorously	3.9	20	78
Bowling	3.4	40	136
Hard			
Playing tennis, doubles	6.7	40	268
Very hard			
No activity	0	0	0
		Total weekly calories	**1,076**

*For 140-pound (63.5-kg) person

Monday
- Walk at lunch—15 minutes
- Walk on break—15 minutes
- Vacuum house—20 minutes

Tuesday
- Walk at lunch—30 minutes

Wednesday
- Tennis after work—45 minutes

Thursday
- Walk at lunch—15 minutes

Friday

No activity

Saturday
- Mow lawn—30 minutes
- Bowling—45 minutes

Sunday
- Walk after lunch—45 minutes

As you can see, most of Flora's activities were at the moderate-intensity level, but she did a combination of things to get her weekly extra 1,000 calories. For most of the activities, she didn't even have to put on workout clothes.

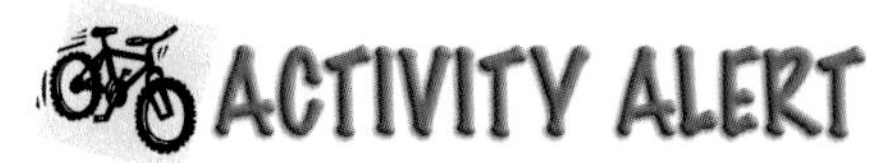

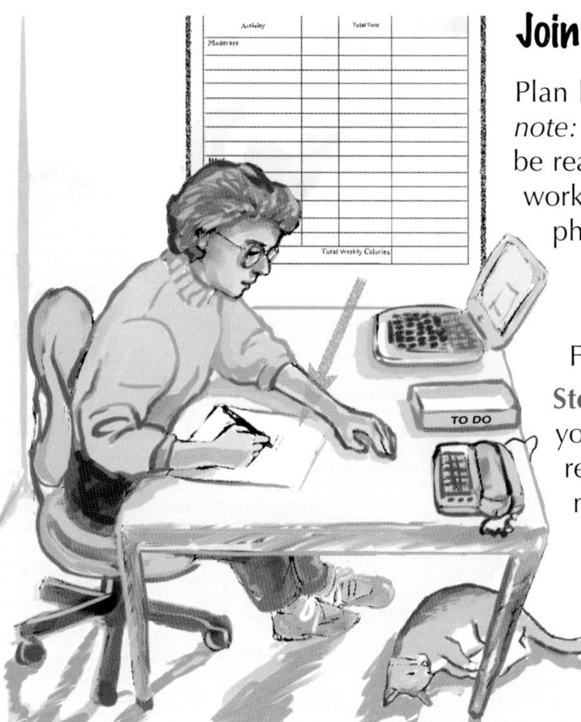

Join the 1,000-Plus Club

Plan how you can burn 1,000 extra calories in a week. *Please note:* At this early stage in the Active Living program, you may not be ready to burn 1,000 or more extra calories a week. Use this worksheet as a guide for when you have sufficiently built up your physical activity level.

Step one. Turn to page 179. This chart shows per minute calorie expenditure for different activities at different weights. Find the column that is closest to your weight.

Step two. Identify the moderate, hard, or very hard activities you could do in one week to increase your physical activity. Be realistic! If you are sedentary, don't decide to run at an eight-minute per mile (1.6 km) pace for 120 minutes. And don't forget those household and yard work chores. They can add quite a few calories to your weekly total.

Step three. Once you have decided on the activities, play around with the amount of time you will spend in each activity. Remember, your total weekly expenditure total should add up to at least 1,000 calories.

Activity	Calories per minute	Total time (minutes)	Total calories (calories per minute × total time)
Moderate			
Hard			
Very hard			
	Total weekly calories		

(continued)

(continued)

Step four. Now plan how you will fit these activities into your week.

Monday

Tuesday

Wednesday

Thursday

Friday

Saturday

Sunday

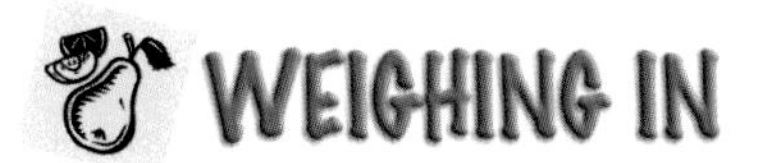

Burning More Calories Than You Eat

What about weight loss? The only way to lose weight is to burn more calories than you eat. You burn most calories in two ways: basic metabolism (energy used for breathing, body processes, beating your heart, etc.) and in physical activity. You don't have much control over your metabolism, but you sure can change your activity level!

As we described in week 2, you have to create a deficit of 3,500 calories (about 500 calories per day) to lose one pound (.5 kg) in a week. This requires your body to call on its energy stores (body fat) to make up the energy deficit. You can create this deficit by eating less, exercising more, or doing a combination of the two. As you have seen from this chapter, there are lots of ways to burn a little or a lot of extra calories. You can modify the intensity, duration, and frequency of your physical activities. In any case, research shows that the best way to maintain a healthy weight is to get active and stay active.

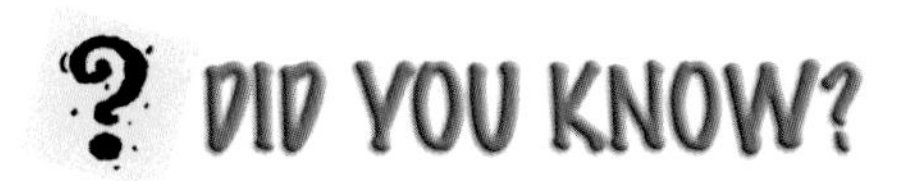

By walking briskly for 10 minutes, you increase your breathing rate from 12 times to 35 times a minute. The amount of air in each breath increases fourfold, from about a pint (.47 L) to one-half gallon (1.9 L). All told, that means your body increases the volume of air you breathe twelvefold while you are walking fast. The result is a strong heart and lungs and improved stamina.

EXPERT ADVICE

Keeping Track of Your Thoughts and Activities

By now we hope we've convinced you that monitoring your activity in minutes or in calories can be a good way to find opportunities and keep track of what you're doing. Scientific studies show that for people who are trying to adopt healthy habits, regular self-monitoring is important. We have designed handy self-monitoring forms to help you keep track of the time you spend doing activities. You can find them on pages 44 and 45 in this chapter. If you haven't become active yet, you can keep track of the time you think about doing activity on the "Keeping Track of Thoughts" form. After all, the more you think about it, the better the chances you'll begin to turn those thoughts into action. Blank copies of the forms are located in appendix D on pages 185-186. Make copies of the forms you need and take them with you every day. We guarantee that by monitoring your activity, you'll greatly increase your chances of success.

KEEPING TRACK OF THOUGHTS

Week of ____________________

Instructions: Use this form to record the number of times you think about doing physical activity. Simply place a check mark (✓) in a box in section 1 each time you *think* about doing some physical activity. If you carried out your thoughts and did the activity you were thinking about, place a check mark (✓) in a box in section 2.

Keeping track of your thoughts about activity can help you start moving toward an active lifestyle.

Section 1 I thought about doing some physical activity.

☐☐☐☐☐☐☐☐☐☐☐☐☐☐☐☐☐☐☐☐☐
☐☐☐☐☐☐☐☐☐☐☐☐☐☐☐☐☐☐☐☐☐
☐☐☐☐☐☐☐☐☐☐☐☐☐☐☐☐☐☐☐☐☐
☐☐☐☐☐☐☐☐☐☐☐☐☐☐☐☐☐☐☐☐☐
☐☐☐☐☐☐☐☐☐☐☐☐☐☐☐☐☐☐☐☐☐
☐☐☐☐☐☐☐☐☐☐☐☐☐☐☐☐☐☐☐☐☐
☐☐☐☐☐☐☐☐☐☐☐☐☐☐☐☐☐☐☐☐☐
☐☐☐☐☐☐☐☐☐☐☐☐☐☐☐☐☐☐☐☐☐

Section 2 I carried out my thoughts and did the activity.

☐☐☐☐☐☐☐☐☐☐☐☐☐☐☐☐☐☐☐☐☐
☐☐☐☐☐☐☐☐☐☐☐☐☐☐☐☐☐☐☐☐☐
☐☐☐☐☐☐☐☐☐☐☐☐☐☐☐☐☐☐☐☐☐
☐☐☐☐☐☐☐☐☐☐☐☐☐☐☐☐☐☐☐☐☐
☐☐☐☐☐☐☐☐☐☐☐☐☐☐☐☐☐☐☐☐☐
☐☐☐☐☐☐☐☐☐☐☐☐☐☐☐☐☐☐☐☐☐
☐☐☐☐☐☐☐☐☐☐☐☐☐☐☐☐☐☐☐☐☐
☐☐☐☐☐☐☐☐☐☐☐☐☐☐☐☐☐☐☐☐☐

KEEPING TRACK OF PHYSICAL ACTIVITY

Week of ______________________________

Instructions: This form is for you to check the amount of time you spend in various activities. After doing an activity, mark the box that best describes the intensity of your activity, moderate or vigorous (see Examples of Activities table on page 46), and its duration. At the end of your week, add the number of minutes checked for each activity category and place it in the "Total minutes" column.

Activity	Intensity level	2 minutes	10 minutes	Total minutes
Garden	Moderate	☐☐☐☐☐ ☐☐☐☐☐ ☐☐☐☐☐	☐☐☐☐☐ ☐☐☐☐☐ ☐☐☐☐☐	
	Vigorous	☐☐☐☐☐ ☐☐☐☐☐ ☐☐☐☐☐	☐☐☐☐☐ ☐☐☐☐☐ ☐☐☐☐☐	
Household	Moderate	☐☐☐☐☐ ☐☐☐☐☐ ☐☐☐☐☐	☐☐☐☐☐ ☐☐☐☐☐ ☐☐☐☐☐	
	Vigorous	☐☐☐☐☐ ☐☐☐☐☐ ☐☐☐☐☐	☐☐☐☐☐ ☐☐☐☐☐ ☐☐☐☐☐	
Leisure	Moderate	☐☐☐☐☐ ☐☐☐☐☐ ☐☐☐☐☐	☐☐☐☐☐ ☐☐☐☐☐ ☐☐☐☐☐	
	Vigorous	☐☐☐☐☐ ☐☐☐☐☐ ☐☐☐☐☐	☐☐☐☐☐ ☐☐☐☐☐ ☐☐☐☐☐	
Occupation	Moderate	☐☐☐☐☐ ☐☐☐☐☐ ☐☐☐☐☐	☐☐☐☐☐ ☐☐☐☐☐ ☐☐☐☐☐	
	Vigorous	☐☐☐☐☐ ☐☐☐☐☐ ☐☐☐☐☐	☐☐☐☐☐ ☐☐☐☐☐ ☐☐☐☐☐	

(continued)

(continued)

Activity	Intensity level	2 minutes	10 minutes	Total minutes
Sports	Moderate	□□□□□ □□□□□ □□□□□	□□□□□ □□□□□ □□□□□	
	Vigorous	□□□□□ □□□□□ □□□□□	□□□□□ □□□□□ □□□□□	
Stairs	Moderate (1 flight up = 10 steps)	□□□□□ □□□□□ □□□□□	□□□□□ □□□□□ □□□□□	
	Vigorous (4 flights up = 2 minutes vigorous work)	□□□□□ □□□□□ □□□□□	□□□□□ □□□□□ □□□□□	
Walking	Moderate	□□□□□ □□□□□ □□□□□	□□□□□ □□□□□ □□□□□	
	Vigorous	□□□□□ □□□□□ □□□□□	□□□□□ □□□□□ □□□□□	

Examples of Activities

Activity	Moderate	Vigorous (hard or very hard)
Garden	Raking, mowing (push), weeding	Shoveling, carrying moderate/heavy loads
Household	Vacuuming carpet, cleaning windows	Moving furniture, shoveling snow
Leisure	Ballroom dancing, fishing from bank (standing or wading)	Pop dancing, backpacking
Occupation	Walking briskly at work	Using heavy tools, fire fighting, loading/unloading truck, laying brick
Sports	Table tennis, golf (no cart), tai chi, Frisbee	Rope jumping, basketball, running, racquetball, soccer
Walking	15-20 minute/mile (1.6 km) pace	Stair climbing, mountain hiking

Purchasing a Step Counter

Another handy way to track your activity is with a step counter. We will introduce you to using the step counter in week 14. To be prepared for this session, in the next few weeks get a step counter at a local sporting goods store or order one from one of the following sources. You should expect to pay $15 to $25.

New Lifestyles
5900 Larson Avenue
Kansas City, MO 64133
888-748-5377
www.digiwalker.com

Accusplit
2290A Ringwood Avenue
San Jose, CA 95131-1718
800-935-1996
www.accusplit.com

Please note: Many pedometers come with extra features such as distance calculation or calories expended. However, these extras are notoriously inaccurate. We recommend you stick with a version that simply counts steps.

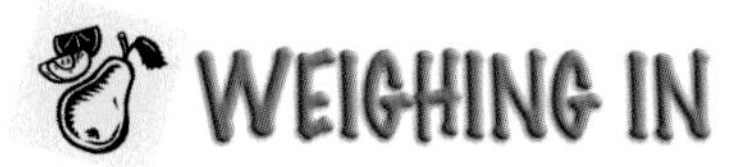

Weight management is a matter of balancing calories taken in via food with calories burned in activity. Here's the amount of activity required for a 160-pound (72.6 kg) person to burn off excess calories equivalent to two popular foods.

	Minutes of activity to burn off calories in	
	Glazed donut (242 calories)	**French fries, large order (400 calories)**
Watching TV	186	308
Walking, 20 min. per mile (1.6 km) pace	58	95
Scrubbing floors	54	89
Dancing (polka, line, country)	42	70
Bicycling, 12 to 14 miles (19.3-22.5 km) per hour	24	39
Running, 9 min. per mile (1.6 km) pace	17	28

A Test You Can Ace

People are often curious about whether they are improving their physical fitness. If you are doing more activity on a regular basis than you were, we can pretty much guarantee that your fitness is improving. But you don't have to take our word for it. Here are two simple tests you can do yourself:

ACTIVITY ALERT

Finding Your Resting Heart Rate

One of the simplest ways to gauge changes in fitness is to track your resting heart rate (beats per minute). As you improve your fitness, your resting heart rate slows. Why? With exercise, your heart gets stronger, so it can pump more with each beat than when you are sedentary. More blood per beat = fewer beats per minute.

Take a moment now, while you're sitting here reading, to take your resting heart rate. Here's how:

The easiest place to find your pulse is on the inside of your wrist, just below your thumb. Place your index and middle fingers lightly against the artery at that location. Chances are you'll feel a little ka-plomp, ka-plomp, ka-plomp. That's your pulse. If you don't feel it, don't panic! Move your fingers until you do. (If you're reading this book, we know your heart is beating!)

Now, using a watch with a second hand, count how many times your heart beats in one minute. Write it down here:

Date	Resting heart rate
______________	______________
______________	______________
______________	______________
______________	______________
______________	______________
______________	______________
______________	______________
______________	______________

Every three to four weeks, measure and record your resting heart rate here. If you're consistently doing physical activity, you'll see it drop. Don't drink caffeinated beverages, eat a heavy meal, or do vigorous exercise three hours before taking your heart rate to ensure an accurate measure.

ACTIVITY ALERT

Taking a Walk Test

Another simple fitness test requires you to map out a route in your neighborhood. It should be at least one-half mile (.8 km) long. Time yourself with a watch that has a second hand as you walk the route *as quickly as you can.* Measure your heart rate 15 seconds immediately after you complete the walk. Record the information in the following chart. Repeat this test periodically to see if you are improving your fitness level. When you can cover the same route in less time or with a lower heart rate it means you've improved your physical fitness. When doing the test follow these simple guidelines:

1. Don't eat a heavy meal or drink caffeinated beverages for at least three hours before the test.
2. Postpone the test if it's extremely cold, hot, or windy.
3. Warm up first by walking slowly for a few minutes.

Route Description

____

____

Date	Time to walk route (minutes and seconds)	Heart rate at end

Some people like to have comprehensive and precise measurements of fitness. For example, you may want to know specifically how much your cardiovascular system is improving, or you may want to track changes in your muscle strength. Body-fat tests can help you learn if you're losing body fat. If you're interested in these or other fitness assessments, contact your local health clubs, Jewish community center, cardiac rehabilitation program, or the exercise program at a nearby university. You should expect to pay between $40 and $75 for a basic fitness assessment.

UP CLOSE & PERSONAL

Jerome participated in our Project *Active* study. Well, we should say he sort of participated. He was assigned to the Lifestyle group and came to the weekly meetings as requested. He was there in body only and, after about eight weeks, stopped coming altogether. We continued to send him the educational materials and tried to reach him by phone on numerous occasions. He was a no-show for most of our assessment visits.

After the study was over and when the scientific papers about the study were being published, we invited the Project *Active* participants back to The Cooper Institute for an appreciation party. Much to our surprise, Jerome showed up, and he looked great! Turns out he was diagnosed with diabetes, and that scared him enough to start changing his lifestyle. He dug out all the Project *Active* materials and worked through them on his own. He told us, "I did everything you told us to do."

What did we learn from Jerome? Even when it seems that people are not interested at the time in changing, they will change when they are ready, as long as they have the tools and information available to them. So even if you're not ready to do all the activities in this book, continue to read through it. You never know when a story or idea might be the trigger to getting you active for a lifetime.

NEED A BOOST?

If you're having a hard time keeping up and meeting your goals, don't worry. Everyone moves forward at his or her own pace, and everybody falters now and then. Try these tips to help you keep on track:

- Review the material in the previous weeks to find ideas that can help you meet your activity goals.
- Find a friend or family member who can encourage you to increase your activity.
- Don't forget: Doing something is better than doing nothing! Try to fit in short bouts of activity whenever you can.
- Find ways to make physical activities fun. Do things you like to do with people you enjoy.
- Physical activity means moving instead of standing, sitting, or lying down. Take a few minutes to think about ways to replace inactive time with moving time.

Chapter Checklist

Before you move on to the next week's activities, make sure you

- Identified activities that are moderate, hard, and very hard
- Estimated your walking pace
- Identified how you can burn 1,000 extra calories per week
- Measured your resting heart rate
- Assessed your fitness level with a walk test
- Ordered a step counter

Why bother calculating the calories you burn? Because energy expenditure is one good way to gauge how active you are. It can also serve as a great way to motivate you to do more than what you have been doing. In the next week, we'll look at how you can use different measures of activity to set goals and monitor your progress.

WEEK **SEVEN**

Setting Goals

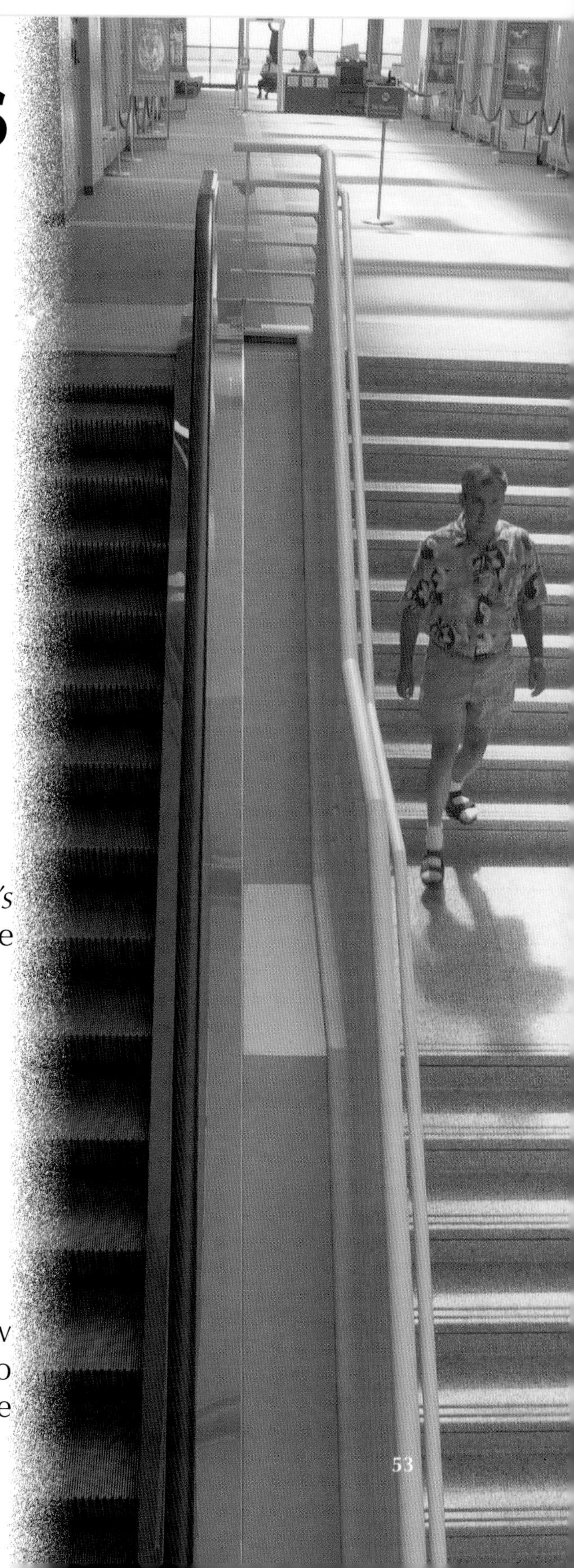

In This Chapter

- Setting goals
- Taking the stairs
- Revisiting self-monitoring

In a famous exchange from Lewis Carroll's *Alice's Adventures in Wonderland,* Alice asked the Cheshire Cat:

> "Would you tell me, please, which way I ought to walk from here?"
>
> "That depends a good deal on where you want to get to," said the Cat.
>
> "I don't much care where," said Alice.
>
> "Then it doesn't matter which way you walk," said the Cat.

The point, of course, is that you have to know where you're going to end up where you want to be. That's just as true when you're trying to change something important in your life. Setting a goal is essential. In fact, experts who study the way people make changes in their lives have found that setting goals is one of the most important keys to success. The clearer your goal, the better the chances you'll reach it.

Measuring Success

When it comes to physical activity, there are several ways to measure success. You can add up the time you spend doing an activity you enjoy, such as walking, and set a goal for increasing your activity time. (Remember the self-monitoring forms we introduced in the last chapter?) Or you can use the Energy Expenditure Chart in appendix C, page 179, to add up how many calories you burn, then shoot for burning more.

The goal you set will help you determine the amount of activity you need to get there. If your goal is to increase cardiovascular fitness and endurance, for instance, it's important to progress toward performing some hard or very hard activities. If your goal is to lose body fat, it may be important to be active at moderate intensities and accumulate more than 30 minutes of activity every day.

UP CLOSE & PERSONAL

Carlos was like many high school athletes. He tried to stay active after he started a career and family, but before long he found himself watching more sports than he played. Once or twice a year he'd run, but it was painful and discouraging. Then Carlos saw an ad on television about Project *Active,* the program we had been running at The Cooper Institute, and he decided to join. He learned about two-minute walks and began adding them to his day. Once he got the hang of that, he began planning his day to include several 10-minute walks. Instead of his usual fast-food lunch, he began to bring a bag lunch and take a 20-minute walk.

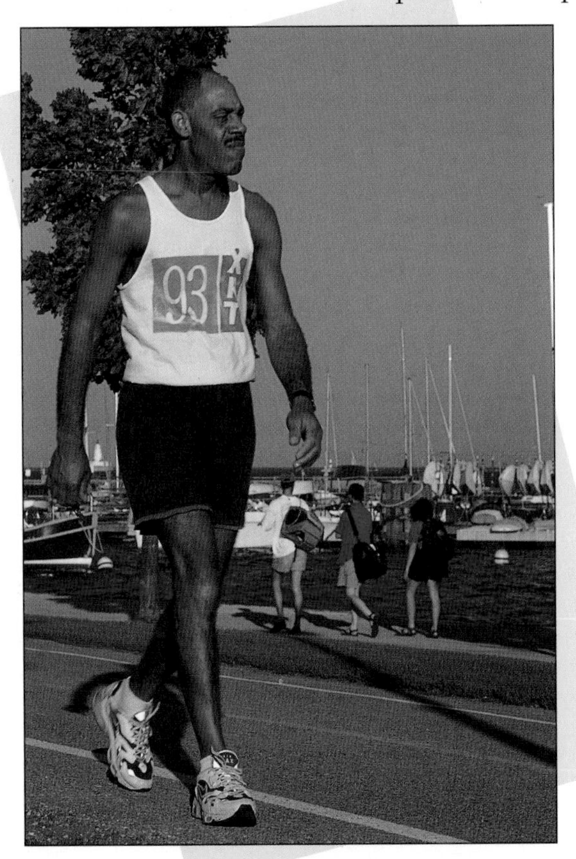

He felt great, but he still missed running. So he set a goal of walking and running in his neighborhood three nights a week. Before long, his goals became more focused. First he wanted to run a 10K race and decided on a race that benefited disabled children. Then he set a goal of playing in the charity basketball event held every May.

Both of these long-term goals helped motivate him to get back in shape. But to meet his long-term goals, he also became specific about short-term goals. During his evening walks and runs, for instance, he would try to add one block each week. Eight weeks later he was running the whole distance. He competed in both the 10K run and the basketball event. While he's had some setbacks along the way, he's managed to make physical activity a regular part of his life again.

EXPERT ADVICE

Tips for Goal Setting

It's not enough simply to say, "I want to become more active." Learning exactly how to set your goal can go a long way toward helping you succeed. Here are three important tips that should help:

1. **Be specific.**

   People who set specific goals do better than people who say, "I'll try to do my best." For example, instead of saying, "This week I'll try to get more exercise," set a specific goal of walking for 15 minutes at every lunch hour and another 15 minutes after dinner.

2. **Set both short-term and long-term goals.**

   A journey of a thousand miles, the Chinese proverb goes, begins with the first step. Short-term goals, in other words, are important if you want to go the distance. If your goal is to walk an hour a day, five days a week, don't expect to reach that goal all at once. A good short-term goal might be to walk for two 15-minute bouts on Saturday, Tuesday, and Thursday, then gradually increase the number of minutes you spend and the number of days a week you walk.

3. **Give yourself feedback.**

   Choose a way to track your progress. You may want to add up the time you spend walking or performing other activities. (If you haven't used the self-monitoring forms, now's the time to give them a try. See pages 184-187.) You may want to use the Energy Expenditure Chart to tally up calories (see page 179). Track your progress day by day and week by week. Chances are you'll begin to see that there are times when you've exceeded your goals and times when you've fallen behind. Everybody does. The value of monitoring your progress is that you'll begin to see the pattern of ups and downs and understand that the downs are only temporary.

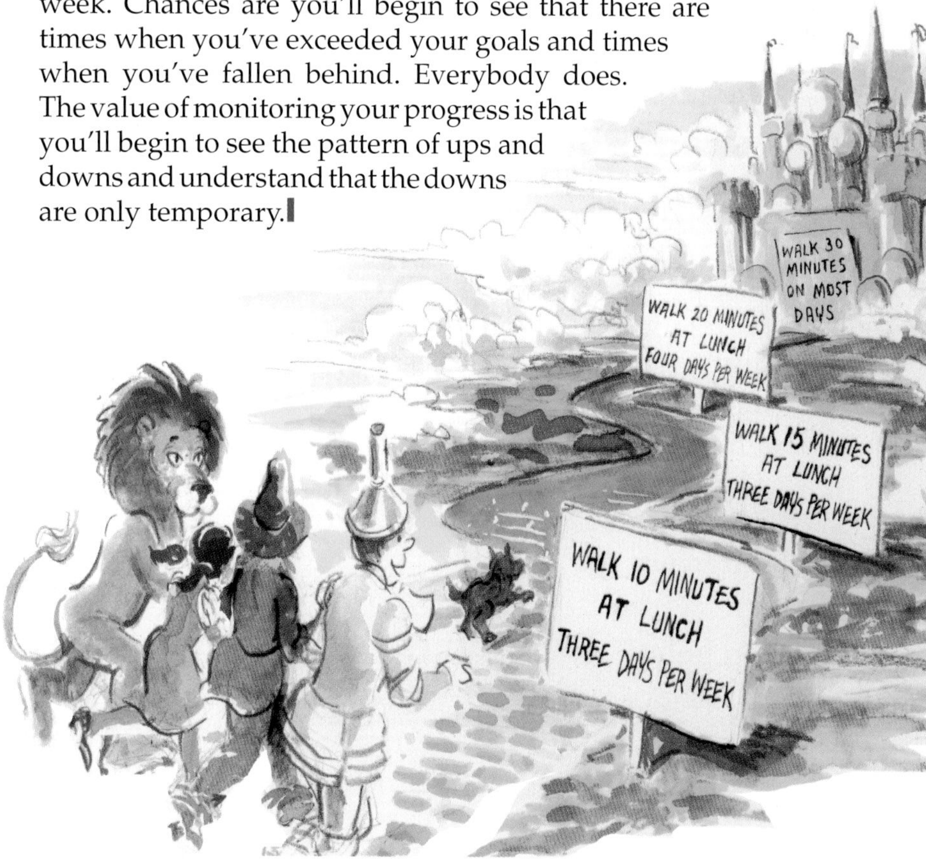

ACTIVITY ALERT

Ready? Set? Goals!

Using the following form, set a goal you intend to meet. Remember to be as specific as you can. It's not enough to say you'll try to walk more often than you have been. Specify how many minutes you plan to walk and when you will do it. Be explicit about how you will monitor your progress. Decide how far into the future your long-term goal should be. (Some people set a one-month goal, others prefer a longer term, such as three months. Be careful not to set a goal so big or so far off that you get discouraged.)

MY GOALS

A short-term goal I can achieve in the next week

____

____

____

____

____

How I plan to monitor my progress

____

____

____

____

____

A long-term goal I hope to achieve by ______________ (date)

____

____

____

____

____

DID YOU KNOW?

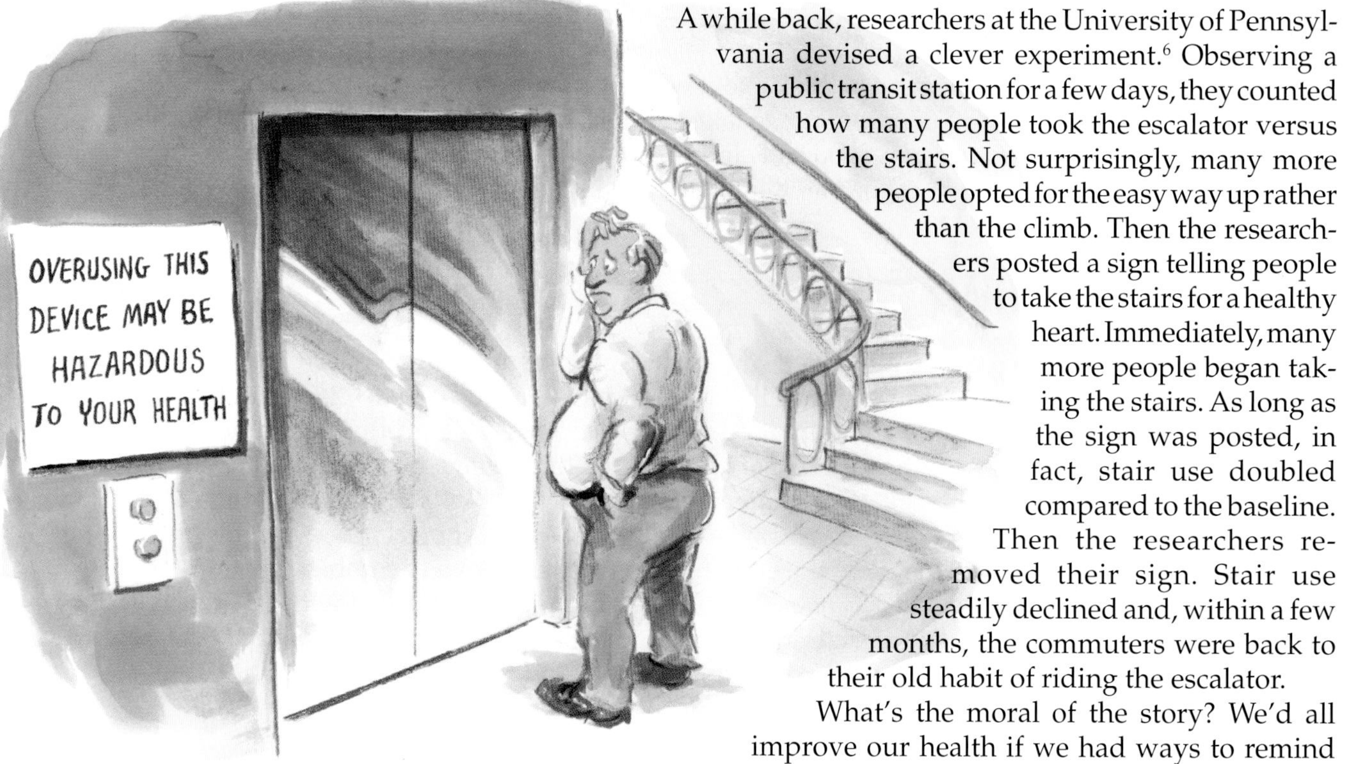

A while back, researchers at the University of Pennsylvania devised a clever experiment.[6] Observing a public transit station for a few days, they counted how many people took the escalator versus the stairs. Not surprisingly, many more people opted for the easy way up rather than the climb. Then the researchers posted a sign telling people to take the stairs for a healthy heart. Immediately, many more people began taking the stairs. As long as the sign was posted, in fact, stair use doubled compared to the baseline. Then the researchers removed their sign. Stair use steadily declined and, within a few months, the commuters were back to their old habit of riding the escalator.

What's the moral of the story? We'd all improve our health if we had ways to remind ourselves about the many potential opportunities we have to be physically active.

EXPERT ADVICE

Step Right Up

By now you've discovered a variety of ways to add brisk walks to your daily routine. Climbing stairs can be a great way to add activity that many people overlook. It's an option many of us face at work, while shopping at the mall, at the airport or bus terminal, and other places we go. Chances are most of us never give it a second thought. Instead of taking the stairs, we take the elevator or escalator.

No wonder. In places such as shopping malls, it's often hard to *find* the staircase. Although the escalators are right in the middle of the building, surrounded by beautiful displays of flowers or merchandise, the staircase is usually in a dim corner, back by the storage area.

Don't let that discourage you. Climbing stairs burns almost 10 times more calories, minute by minute, than riding up the elevator or escalator. Stair climbing burns two to three times as many calories as walking the equivalent amount of time, because with each step up you lift your body weight (plus whatever you're carrying). Climbing stairs burns as many calories per minute as jogging, playing racquetball or tennis, or hiking with a heavy backpack. And you'll give your leg and buttock muscles a little tune-up—not bad for a few flights of stairs.

ACTIVITY ALERT

Taking the Stairs

Take a moment to think about where you go and what you do during the day. Are there opportunities to take the stairs instead of an escalator or elevator? Is there a staircase you can climb when you take a break at work? Make a list of opportunities for stair climbing in your daily life.

DID YOU KNOW?

In a recently published study, researchers at the University of Ulster and the Queen's University of Belfast[7] conducted a study with 22 inactive young women who were divided into two groups. One group maintained their usual activities. The other added stair climbing every day. Each day during the first week, they climbed a single staircase with 199 steps, which took approximately 135 seconds. The second week, they climbed two flights of stairs each day. By the end of seven weeks, they were climbing six flights of stairs distributed over the course of each day. Compared with the inactive women, the stair climbers increased their fitness, lowered their total cholesterol level, and improved the ratio of good to bad cholesterol! That's a big payoff for less than 14 minutes of stair climbing each day.

UP CLOSE & PERSONAL

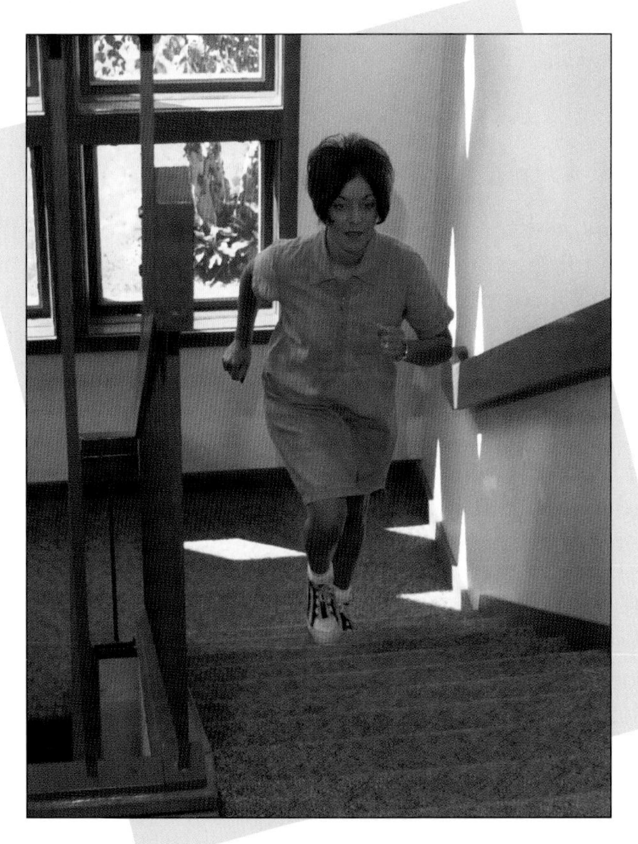

Elena traveled frequently to Central and South America in her work as a buyer for a leading import company. When she was home she managed to stick to her activity plan. But when she was on the road she often found it difficult to be active.

One day a colleague told her that he'd had the same problem until he realized that stairwells in hotels were a perfect way to get a quick workout almost anywhere. The next time Elena traveled, she asked the hotel manager for a room on the fourth floor. In the morning, in the late afternoon, and again in the evening, she climbed up and down the stairs twice. Now she has made stair climbing a regular part of her travel plans.

DID YOU KNOW?

Anyone who lights up a cigarette these days knows they're doing themselves and those around them real harm. All of us know that we'd be better off having a piece of fruit for dessert than helping ourselves to a fat slice of chocolate decadence (unless it's a special occasion, of course). But taking the escalator instead of the stairs? Most of us never even pause. We never think, uh-oh, if I take the elevator instead of the stairs I'm likely to raise my risk of heart disease or die young.

However, over time, the cumulative effect of inactivity *is* harmful. Indeed, the epidemic of inactivity in the United States may be more harmful to our health than an overrich diet. It may be just as harmful as smoking. In a study at The Cooper Institute, for instance, we followed over 32,000 people for eight years. People whose only risk factor was low fitness were significantly more likely to die prematurely than those who had high blood pressure, high cholesterol, or a smoking habit, but who were at least moderately fit. In other words, moderate fitness—achievable by doing moderate-intensity activities on most days—can help counteract even well-known risk factors for disease.[8]

Chapter Checklist

Before you move on to the next week's activities, make sure you

- Made a list of short-term and long-term goals
- Made plans to monitor your progress
- Identified at least one opportunity to climb stairs during the day

By the end of this week, you will have a clear set of goals in mind *and* you'll be taking the stairs more often than you have before. In the next week, we'll look at getting the support you need to meet those goals.

WEEK **EIGHT**

Enlisting Support

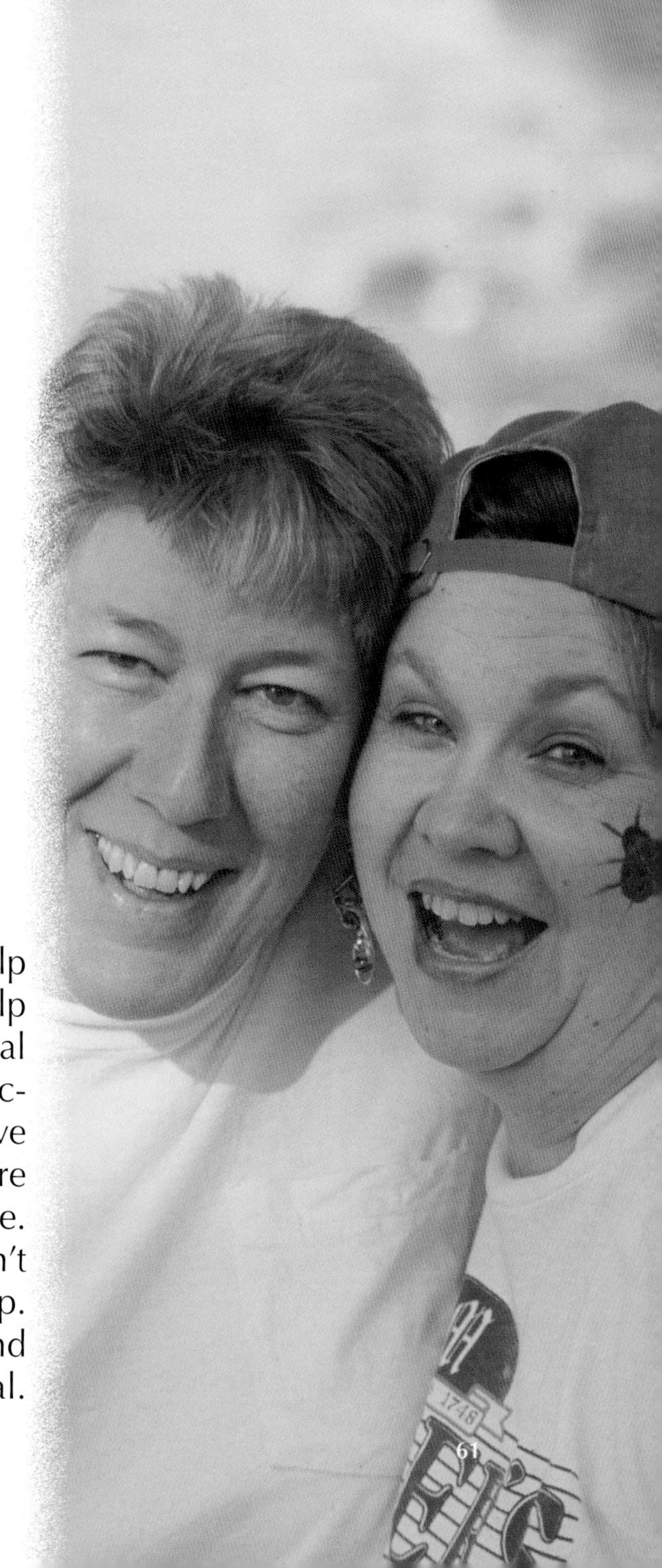

In This Chapter

- Listing the kinds of support you need
- Identifying key sources of support
- Spotting people who may make things difficult
- Learning how to ask for help

As the Beatles once sang, "I get by with a little help from my friends." The truth is, we can all use help once in a while. Research shows that social support is a crucial ingredient to making a successful change in your life. The more supportive your family, friends, and coworkers are, the more likely you are to succeed in any kind of change. But if you don't have support at home, don't despair. There are other places to turn for help. Knowing the kind of support you need—and where to find it—can help you stick to your goal.

EXPERT ADVICE

Finding the Support You Need

There are all kinds of support and all kinds of people who can offer it to you. Here are some examples:

- **Listening support.** This kind of help usually comes from people who listen to your triumphs and troubles without giving advice or making judgments about your thoughts or behavior. In other words, they're good sounding boards.
- **Shared experience support.** This help comes from someone who's in the same boat as you are, knows what you're going through, and can sympathize with your feelings. People who've had similar experiences can often offer helpful suggestions. Just knowing you're not the only one who has gone through something can be reassuring.
- **Technical support.** This usually comes from a person with real expertise who can offer useful tips and good advice. Health professionals are a good source of information. So are books, videos, newspapers, magazines, or television. Be careful, though. Not all information is accurate or well-balanced. Some sources promote magic potions or products (the tip-off is when they ask you to send in $29.95 for some newfangled exercise device or diet breakthrough). Others offer quick fixes that really *are* too good to be true.

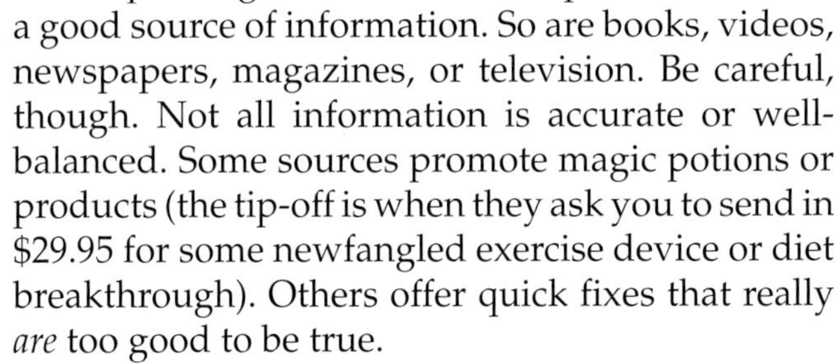

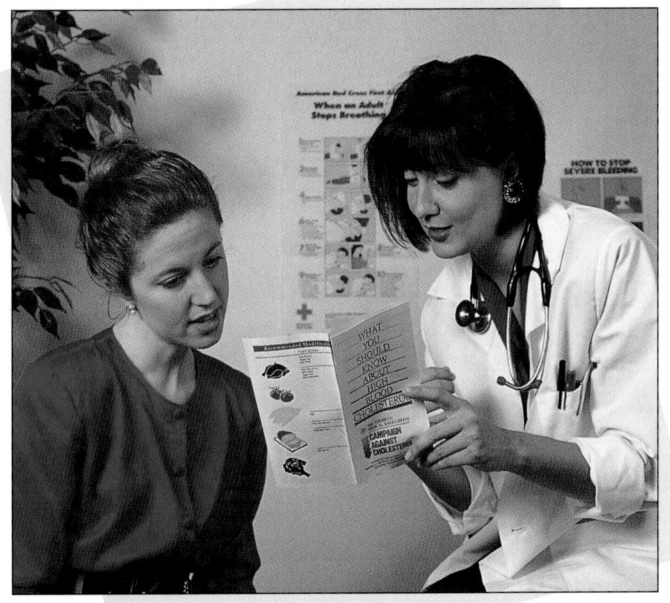

Health professionals can often offer expert and practical advice.

- **Partnering support.** This is offered by that special someone who's willing to join you on your morning walk or your bike ride after work. A walking or cycling partner makes it easier to get out of bed on those mornings when you just don't feel like it. When someone else is depending on you for moral support, it's hard to blow it off and say no. Someone who offers to be a partner can give you that initial push you need to make activity a regular habit.
- **Motivational support.** This kind of help comes from somebody who can pump up your determination or confidence—a cheerleader type who is upbeat, energetic, and enthusiastic.
- **Emotional support.** This is offered by someone who knows you and how you're feeling. Your happiness and well-being are all that matter to someone who offers genuine emotional support. A casual friend or coworker may offer good listening support, but real emotional support usually comes from a close friend or relative.
- **Practical support.** This includes any help that makes it easier for you to succeed in making a lasting change in your life. It may be a spouse who takes on a few household chores to give you time for your walk after dinner or a grandparent nearby who can sit with the kids while you go to a dance class.

UP CLOSE & PERSONAL

Over the last two years, Marilyn often tried to increase her activity, and usually she did—for a week or two. Then work or family got in the way and her resolve fizzled.

Then she noticed that her neighbor Carol walked every morning before breakfast. When Marilyn asked if she could join her, Carol said she would be delighted. She was happy for the company. Marilyn was glad to have someone to motivate her. Now, even on days when she's rushed or not in the mood, she knows Carol is waiting, and she's not about to let her down. This is a great example of partnering support. The fact that Carol and Marilyn became better friends was the spoonful of sugar that made the exercise pill go down.

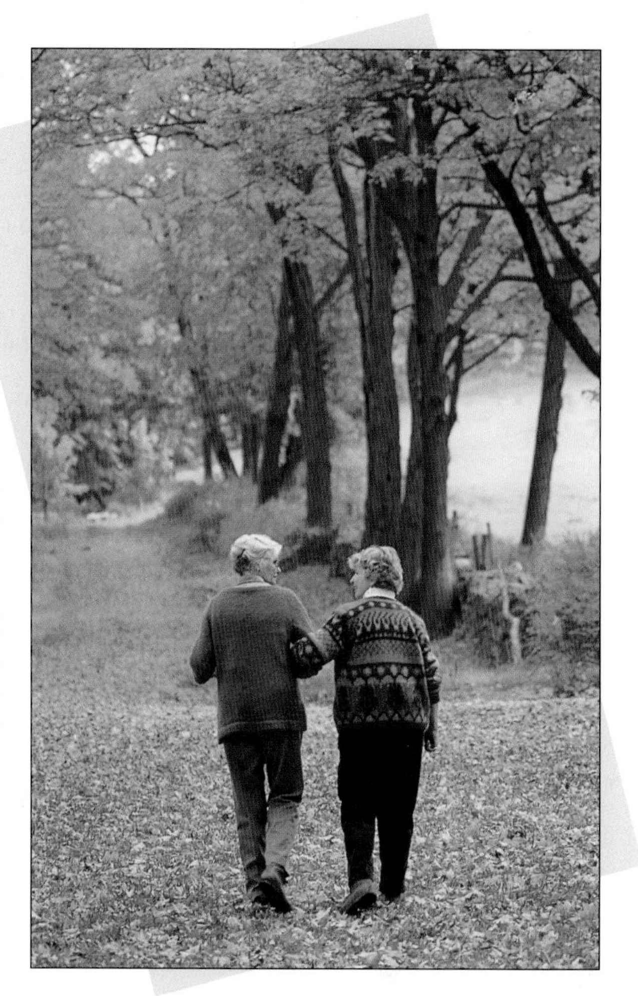

Who Can You Turn To?

Not all of us need all these kinds of support all the time. At first, you may need shared experience or informational support to help you get past the early hurdles. Later you may get more out of motivational or practical support to help you stick to your goals.

Remember, no single person is likely to offer all these forms of support (that person would have to be a saint). One person may be better at listening; another may be better at discussing shared experiences. Don't count on your spouse or significant other to be all things to you. You could put too much strain on your friendship or relationship.

Who to turn to? Support can come from many people around you, your kids, for instance. Look for opportunities to play with them, take a walk together, or engage in other active pursuits. Your spouse or significant other can also help. An early morning or after dinner walk is a great way for you to spend time together, talk over the events of the day, and get in some activity.

Chances are your friends, neighbors, or coworkers are other good people to turn to for support, especially anyone who can offer shared experiences or is willing to lace up a pair of walking shoes and join you.

DID YOU KNOW?

In a survey of 1,000 non-exercisers commissioned by the President's Council on Physical Fitness and Sports and the Sporting Goods Manufacturers Association, 59 percent said they would like to exercise more.[9] What did two out of five say would be the biggest motivator? A spouse or significant other who supported and encouraged them. Even better, said the respondents, was a friend or relative to exercise with them.

UP CLOSE & PERSONAL

From her experience with making other changes in her life, Sharita knew she worked better with other people around to support and encourage her. She also knew, from involvement in her local church, that there were many other women in the community who were looking for a way to increase their physical activity.

After the first few weeks in our program, Sharita took the initiative and organized a walking club with other women from her church. They began to meet in the evenings to walk around a local high school track. Whenever a woman missed a session, she had to put a dollar in the kitty. At the end of three months, the walkers who showed up most often got to share the money from the kitty. The real reward, of course, was enjoyed by all of them: a little extra motivation to help them reach their goal to increase their activity. This is a great example of emotional, motivational, and partnering support, all rolled into one.

Just Ask!

How can you find the support you need? Just ask! Many of us are uneasy asking for help, either because we fear rejection or we see it as a sign of weakness. In fact, everyone needs help from time to time, and most people are happy to offer it. When you ask for support, be open and candid. Explain why you're trying to become more active and why the support of people around you is so important. Be specific about what would help most. It's not enough to say to your kids, "Hey, how about cutting me a little slack?" Chances are you'll get more help by telling them exactly what they can do to help, for example cooking dinner or cleaning up the kitchen after dinner so you have time for a half-hour walk.

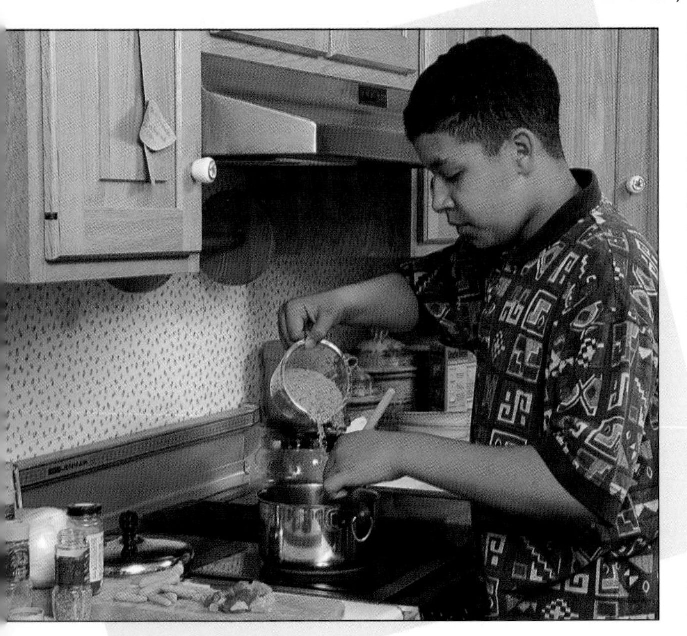

Ask your family members to do something specific to help free up time for you to exercise.

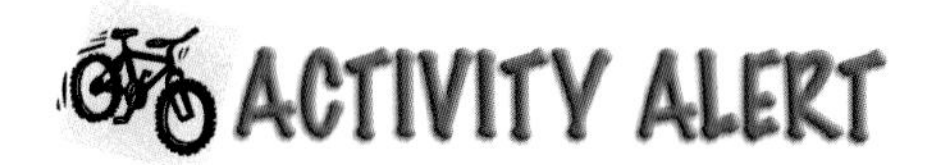

Recruiting Your Support Troops

Use the form on this page to recruit your supporters. First, take a moment to think about the things that still get in your way, such as lack of time or not feeling motivated. Be as specific as possible about the practical or emotional support that would help you overcome these barriers. Then think about the best people to turn to for the help you need. After you've put together your list of supporters, make a plan to talk to them.

MY SUPPORT TROOPS

What do I need help with?	Who could help me?	How could they help?	How could I reward them for helping me?
Example Remembering to fit in physical activity during the day	My coworker Susan or my friend Charles	Call me once a day to check on how much activity I have gotten.	Every two weeks,take him or her to a movie.

ACTIVITY ALERT

Solo or With a Group

Some people like to go it alone, others love company. If you thrive on companionship, take a few minutes this week to check out activity clubs in your area. Most places have groups that get together to walk, run, cycle, skate, hike, swim, or dance (ballroom, country and western, tap, swing, etc.). Call the recreation department or check the local newspaper. Use the blank lines below to put together a list of what you discover. If you don't find what you're looking for, consider starting your own group of lunchtime walkers or after-work bikers by posting a message at the office cafeteria, at your church, or the local recreation center.

Would you just as soon be on your own? That's great. Some people like to use activities such as walking as a way to relax and think. Still, consider turning to people around you for support and encouragement. Tell a friend or family member about your plan to become active and how you hope to carry it out. Knowing that this person will ask you now and then, "How's your bike riding or walking going?" will help keep you motivated. If you're a go-it-alone person, use the blanks below to write down the names of two or three people who could encourage you:

____

____

____

UP CLOSE & PERSONAL

When Barry joined our program, inactivity wasn't his only worry. After a painful divorce, he was having trouble with his teenage son, who felt angry and confused. A week after he began a walking regimen, Barry decided to invite his son to join him for a brisk walk before dinner. The boy was reluctant, but he finally agreed. Because he didn't know how to fix dinner for himself, he figured he had no choice. Their walks were quiet at first, full of "I don't know," and "whatever," but after a while they began talking. Once they broke the ice, their conversations became more intimate. They began to talk about their feelings about the divorce and what lay ahead. Adding a simple activity to family life had provided a benefit Barry never expected.

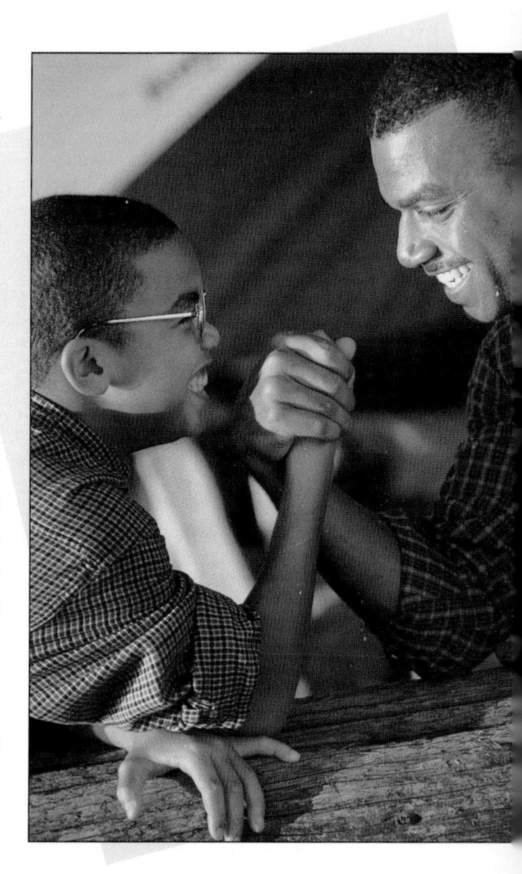

Exercising with family members can bring unexpected benefits.

Chapter Checklist

Before you move on to the next week's activities, make sure you

- Identified two or three people who can support you in your effort to become active
- Specified the kind of help you need most
- Identified ways to help your support troops in return

If you're like many people in our programs, you've had your ups and downs. You've met your goals—maybe even exceeded them—during some weeks. Other weeks you've barely gotten off the sofa. Don't be discouraged. If you've stuck with us this far, you've also been learning that you can have ups and downs and still be making progress. We hope that seeking the support of family and friends will help you reach your physical activity goals. In the coming week, we'll look at ways to boost your confidence.

EXPERT ADVICE

Beware the Exercise Saboteurs

Unfortunately, you may encounter people who try to discourage you or even sabotage your plans to make a lifestyle change. If those around you are indifferent or actively opposed to your efforts to become active, you'll find it harder to succeed than if you have the support you need.

Why would anyone want to scuttle your plans? Change is threatening, especially to those we're closest to. A spouse or significant other may interpret your decision to become physically active as a criticism of him or her or as dissatisfaction with the relationship. Your coworkers may feel threatened by your resolution to increase your activity, especially if they feel uneasy or guilty about their own inactivity.

Lack of support can take many forms. A spouse may complain about the time you spend exercising or throw roadblocks in your path in hopes of derailing you. Your boss may try to sabotage your lunchtime walks by scheduling meetings at noon. Even the best-intentioned friends can make it tough. They may want you to go to lunch with them, and they'll pressure you in friendly ways that could be harder to resist than outright opposition.

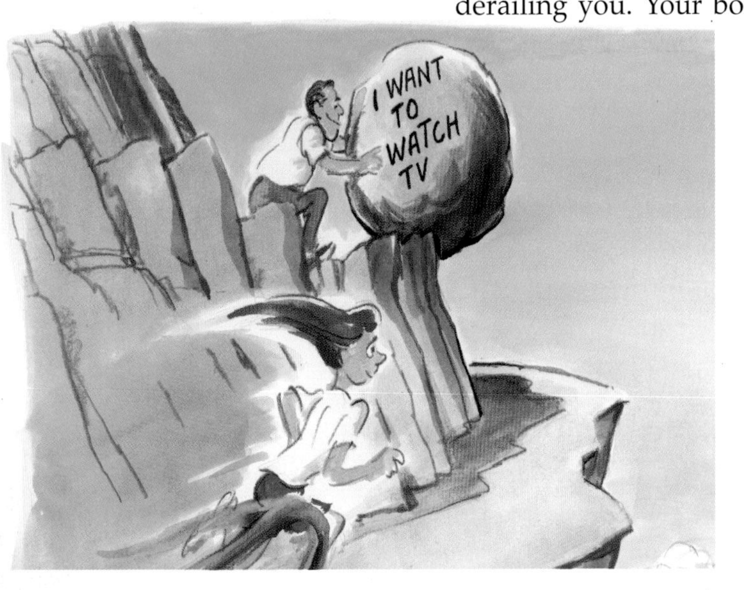

What can you do if you meet opposition? Be open and positive, but also firm about your determination. Reassure your spouse or significant other that increasing your activity doesn't threaten your relationship. Better yet, try to involve him or her in your activities. The same goes for your boss or coworkers. Explain why your decision to become active is important to you and why you need help making it happen. Be friendly and accommodating. If you don't want to go to lunch with coworkers today, for instance, take a rain check for another day.

UP CLOSE & PERSONAL

Tony joined our program out of concern for not only his health but also his family's health. He was particularly worried about his wife's inactivity and the message their inactivity conveyed to their kids. He had his heart set on having his wife walk with him. When she refused, he became discouraged. It was more than just a refusal. When he persisted in trying to persuade her to join him, she began to ridicule his efforts. Fortunately, he recognized that he was only making things worse by insisting, so he turned elsewhere for support. He began talking to his coworkers at the warehouse about walking at lunchtime. He found several who agreed to walk around the nearby mall with him. (It turned out that they had also been looking for ways to become active.) Of course, he still hopes his wife will eventually join him, but his activity no longer depends solely on her support.

WEEK **NINE**

Gaining Confidence

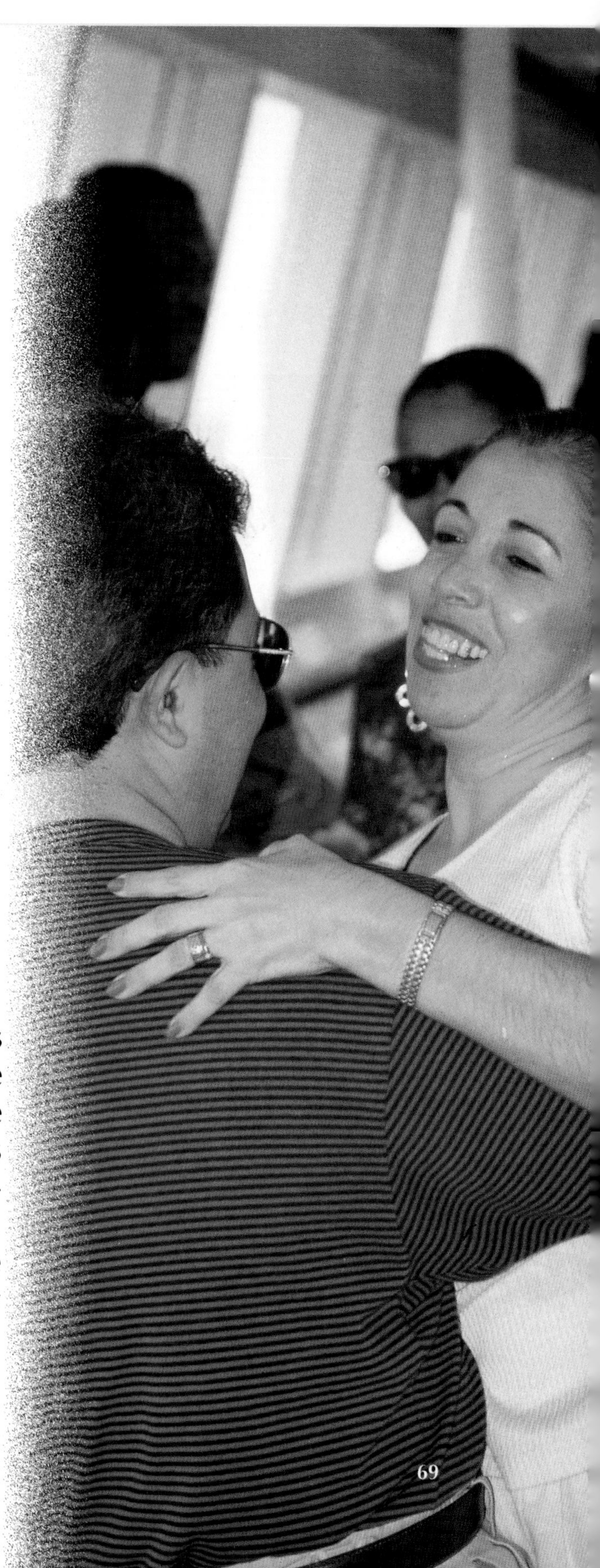

In This Chapter

- Replacing negative messages with positive strategies
- Identifying errands that can become opportunities for activity
- Revisiting the stages of change

We've all heard that little voice in our heads that says, "I can't." On other occasions, we've heard a different, confident, self-assured voice say, "Of course I can. *No problem.*" In this chapter we'll look at ways to silence the negative voice and replace it with a positive one. Along the way we'll discover the confidence that comes from turning "I can't" into "I know I can."

EXPERT ADVICE

Countering Negative Arguments

Let's start by considering a few of the top 10 reasons *not* to get up and do something active. Some we've talked about before. At least one is probably a reason you've used yourself. For every one of the negatives, there's a good counterargument.

"I'm Too Tired to Move"

We've all used this excuse as a reason for flopping on the couch and not moving for the rest of the evening, but consider this: physical activity usually makes people feel energized. Many volunteers in our program reported feeling invigorated after walking or taking a bicycle out for a spin. If you're too tired to move, the best remedy is usually to get up and *move.*

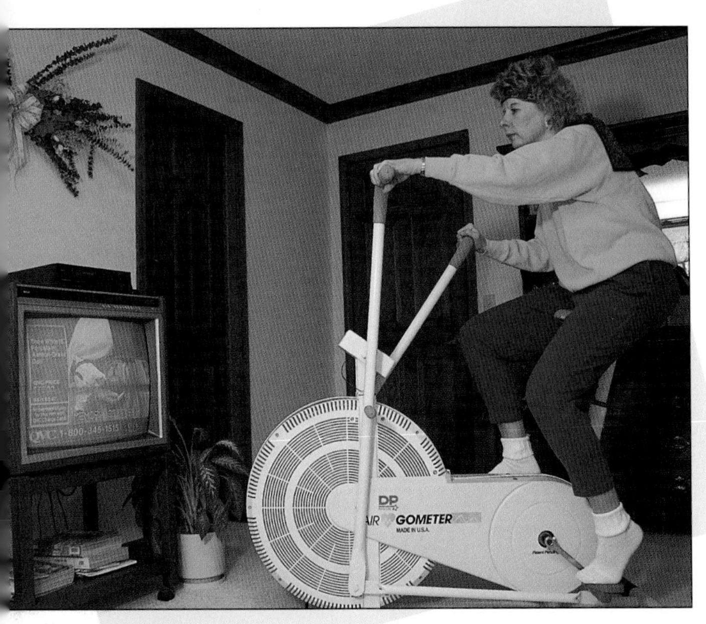

You can get a good workout in the privacy of your home, even by exercising during commercials!

"It's Been a Stressful Day and I'm in a Rotten Mood"

We've all been there. Stress can wear most of us down. But the worst thing you can do is sit and fret. Dozens of studies have shown that physical activity is a great way to relieve stress and blow off the frustrations of the day. Most people report feeling happy and relaxed after a game of tennis, a soothing swim, or a walk around the neighborhood. Another plus: You'll experience the satisfaction of meeting your activity goal.

"I Have Way Too Much Work to Do"

It may seem that way, but before you scuttle your plan to be active, consider this: taking a short activity break could improve your productivity. When people work without a break, productivity usually begins to slump. Get up from your desk for a five-minute walk, climb a few flights of stairs, take a walk around the block at lunch, and chances are you'll return feeling focused and full of energy to get the job done.

"It's Too Cold (or Hot or Rainy or Snowy) to Go Outside"

Fair enough. That's why it's important to have a backup plan. If you don't feel like walking outside, consider walking in the mall. If the weather is so bad you'd rather not drive to a mall, find a few things to do around the house, such as simple calisthenics, jumping rope, or some heavy-duty housecleaning. However, if cold or rainy weather is a fact of life where you live, you can put together the clothes you need to brave the elements. Waterproof warm-up suits can keep you dry. Down jackets, gloves, and hats keep you warm. Once you start moving, you'll hardly notice the cold wind.

"I Want to Watch My Favorite TV Program Tonight"

Go ahead. Enjoy. Watching your favorite TV show, however, doesn't have to mean not being active. Some volunteers in our programs used a rowing machine or a stationary bike while watching television. Others made a point of getting up during the commercials to stretch, take a quick walk, climb the stairs, or do a few calisthenics. Another strategy is to schedule a 10-minute walk before and after your favorite program. Right there you've tallied up 20 minutes. If your goal is to get one-half hour of activity every day, another 10 minutes should be easy to find.

Our point is simple: for every good reason not to be active, there's an even better reason to get up and do something. One great way to build confidence and encourage yourself is to create a positive message to counteract those negative thoughts that sometimes get in your way.

ACTIVITY ALERT

Confidence Building

Here's a list of the problems that keep people from being active and can tear down the confidence you have been working hard to build. Countering these problems can help you solve them. Better still, overcoming problems builds confidence.

ACCENTUATING THE POSITIVE

Read the negative messages below. Circle the ones that you've said to yourself sometimes. Then write down at least one counterargument that accentuates the positive.

1. I don't want to do anything when I feel tired or down in the dumps.

____

____

____

____

2. I don't know how to get started.

____

____

____

____

(continued)

(continued)

ACCENTUATING THE POSITIVE

3. I don't have anyone to be active with me.

4. I can't find the time in my busy schedule.

5. I'm going on vacation.

6. I'm having a personal crisis.

7. I just can't remember to exercise.

8. I'm too sore from the last time.

9. My family and friends don't support me.

10. I haven't been feeling well all week.

11. I'm discouraged because I never seem to reach my activity goal.

12. I don't like to be active in public because I'm embarrassed by the way I look.

(continued)

(continued)

If we've missed the negative message that gets in your way, write it down. How can you replace the negative with a positive?

____

____

____

____

UP CLOSE & PERSONAL

As a kid, Brenda could never live up to her parents' high expectations for her. Now, at 35, she still heard their voices in her head saying, "Why can't you try a little harder?" and "You'll never be a success if this is the best you can do." Those negative messages were especially loud whenever she looked at herself in the mirror and saw an overweight and out-of-shape reflection staring back at her. Now and then she'd try to take up an activity such as walking or swimming. But something always got in the way.

When Brenda joined Project *Active*, she'd all but given up on becoming an active person. At first, all our work didn't shake that pessimistic idea. Then Brenda sat down with a sheet of paper and looked squarely at the barriers that kept getting in her way. One problem was that she couldn't find the support she needed. Another was that she sometimes felt too tired and sad. A third reason was that her schedule sometimes became so hectic she didn't have time.

For each barrier, she came up with a counterstatement that built confidence rather than discouragement. Sure she sometimes had trouble finding support from her husband, but she also knew that when she set her mind to it, she could do it on her own.

Yes, her moods sometimes got in the way, but then all she had to do was remind herself that getting out and walking briskly often lifted her mood and made her feel happy. True, her schedule at work was sometimes crazy, but with a little planning, she told herself, she could always find 10 minutes here, 10 minutes there. Gradually, each time a negative message threatened to overwhelm her resolve, Brenda reminded herself of the positive countermessage. Each time she countered the negative message and did some activity, her confidence increased.

Celebrating Small Victories

Confidence comes from setting a goal, making a plan, and achieving it. Unfortunately, we often neglect to celebrate our own victories. That's especially true for people who have tried and failed before. All they can see is failure.

During the past few weeks, we hope, you've been able to meet your personal goals more than once. Over time, those small steps can add up to real success. Take a moment now and review what you've accomplished so far. Look back over the previous chapters and the goals you've set for yourself. Sure, you may not have scored 100 percent each week. Few people do. No matter. Every small advance means progress.

ACTIVITY ALERT

My Accomplishments

In the following space, write three things you've accomplished so far—things you're proud of. Maybe you met your goal of 30 minutes a day for an entire week. Maybe you sat down and made a plan for the first time. Maybe your big breakthrough was finally recognizing the negative voice that always talks you into failure. That alone is an important step toward success.

1.____

2.____

3.____

Now that you've completed the list, pat yourself on the back for a job well done.

DID YOU KNOW?

A century ago, most people couldn't help but get plenty of exercise. Household chores such as washing, cleaning, and ironing required hard physical labor. Working on a farm or in a factory meant working up a sweat. People walked to town and back instead of jumping into a car. In countless ways, the labor-saving devices of the 20th century have vastly improved the way we live and work. Factories have become wonders of automation. Thanks to farm machinery, farmers can create high yields that feed the earth's burgeoning population. Cars and planes have put once remote or inaccessible places within reach.

However, recently researchers have begun to see an unexpected drawback. The human body, it turns out, is built to be active. Our muscles need to lift and pull to remain strong. Our hearts need to beat fast once in a while to stay healthy. Our lungs need to exert themselves to promote stamina. Without physical activity, we're learning, the risk of developing chronic diseases begins to climb.

No one is suggesting we turn back the wheels of progress, but the latest findings on physical activity and health make it clear that we must find new ways to incorporate activity into everyday life.

ACTIVITY ALERT

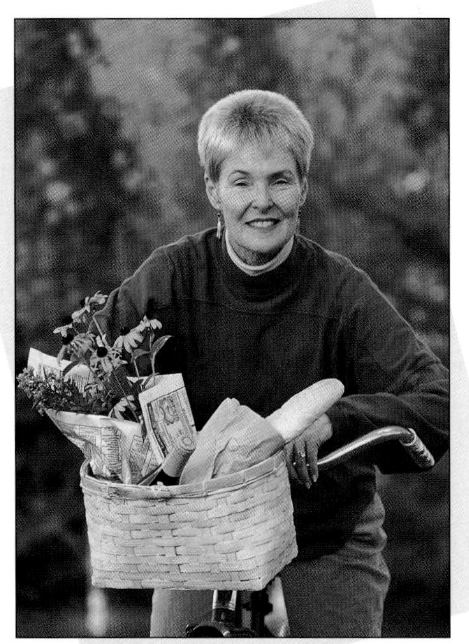
Which of your errands can you turn into physical activities?

Turning Errands Into Activity

Whether we're picking up groceries for dinner, stopping by the post office, or going to the bank, most of us run at least a few errands every day. Unfortunately, we don't really run. We don't even walk. We drive or take the bus. We wait in line. We get back in the car and drive home. Such day-to-day errands represent great opportunities for increasing your activity. All it takes is a little planning. For starters, make a list of the typical errands you run during the week. Some you may do every day, others just once a week. Include everything that comes to mind.

A WEEK'S WORTH OF ERRANDS

1. ______________________________

2. ______________________________

3. ______________________________

4. ______________________________

5. ______________________________

Now look over the list and select two or three errands that, with a little tweaking, you could turn into physical activities. Let's say you typically drive to the grocery store, even though it's only five blocks from home. Walking there and back is a great opportunity to add 15 minutes of exercise and burn around 75 calories. Sure there are times when it's not practical to walk, especially when you have to pick up a lot of groceries, but if you need just a few things for dinner, walking is a great alternative.

The same goes for errands to the bank or post office. Live too far to walk? Then select a place several blocks from your destination to park the car or get off the bus and walk the rest of the way. If you can, choose a path that's pleasant and interesting to add another incentive. Over the next week, carry out your plan to turn a few errands into activities. If you keep a daily to-do list, add a star to the errands you've selected to serve as a reminder.

ACTIVITY ALERT

How Far Have You Come?

It's the end of week 9 and time to look back at your readiness to change to see how far you've come. No need to introduce the Readiness to Change flow chart. It's old hat by now. Answer honestly. After you're done, look back to weeks 2 and 5 to see if your answers are different now.

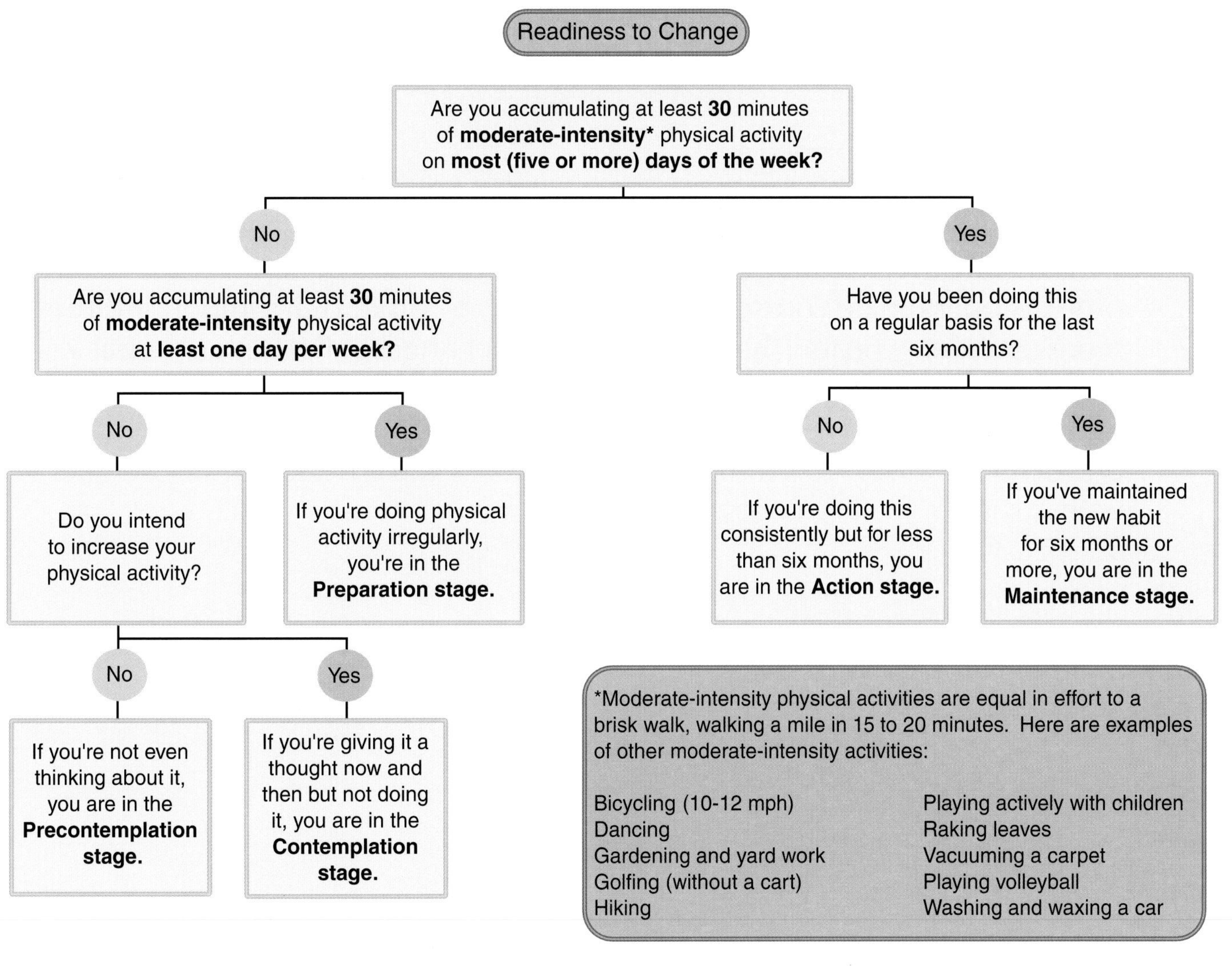

If you've moved a step ahead in the stages of change, congratulations. Treat yourself to something special this weekend as a reward. Even if you haven't changed your stage, chances are you're still making progress. Moving between stages often takes time. Some people stay in the preparation stage for several months before they move into action. It takes six months of being in the action stage before you can graduate to maintenance. Don't get discouraged. Remember, progress toward your goal isn't often in a straight line forward. For every two steps forward, there is sometimes a step back. As long as you hold to your commitment and remind yourself why it matters to you to become active, you'll do fine. If you need more help, look at the "Stages of Change" tips in appendix B.

Chapter Checklist

Before you move on to the next week's activities, make sure you

- Identified negative messages that keep you from being physically active
- Listed your important accomplishments so far
- Turned at least two errands into opportunities for activity
- Completed the Readiness to Change form that charts your progress

This week, you've noted some negative messages you sometimes give yourself and tried replacing them with positive messages. You've also taken time to congratulate yourself on how far you've come. That's important. The more confident you feel that you can make a change for the better, the easier it will be to make activity a lifelong habit. Feeling confident about yourself as an active person will also inspire you to try new forms of activity. That's one of the best ways to stay motivated. Next week we'll take a little breather with a short refresher course.

WEEK **TEN**

Strengthening the Foundation

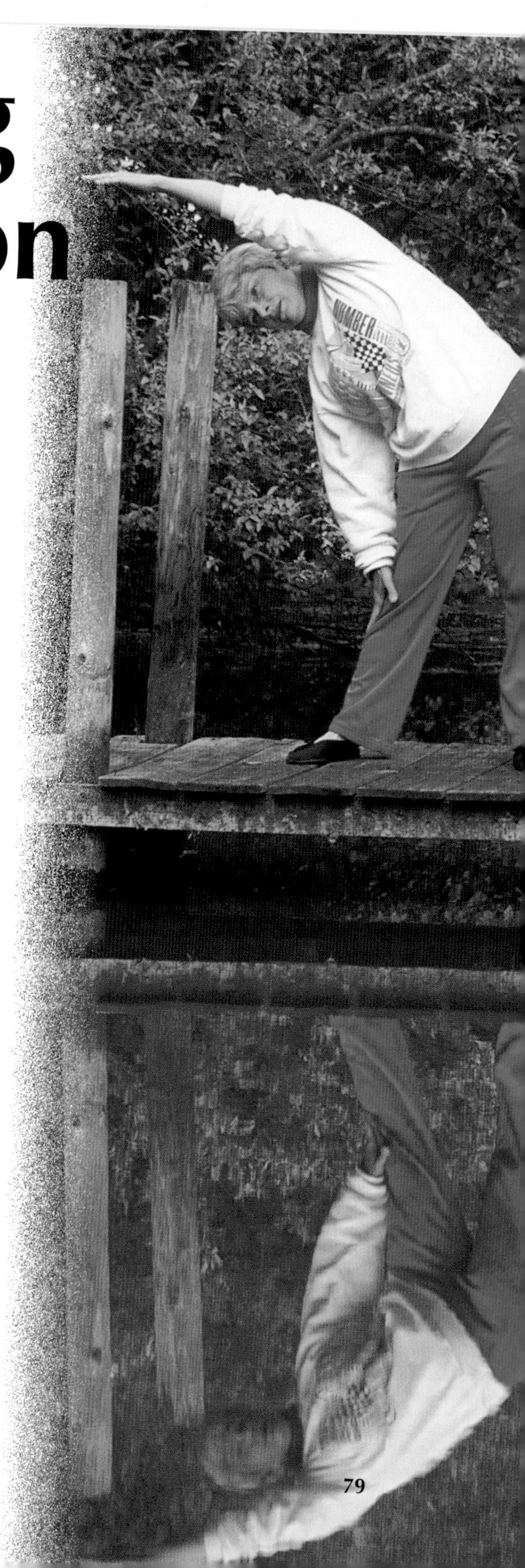

In This Chapter

- Revisiting earlier activities
- Learning a few stretching techniques
- Testing your knowledge

Chances are you've already experienced some important changes in your life. Maybe you've begun to feel more confident about being active than you used to be. Maybe you're feeling more energetic. Perhaps you've even trimmed down by losing a little body fat and adding some muscle. Even if you've only strengthened your commitment to change, that's important progress.

This week we will look back at how far you've come and do a quick refresher course on what we've covered so far. We will also offer you a chance to try a few more everyday activities that you might enjoy.

Revisiting Earlier Territory

Nobody learns everything the first time around. The process of becoming an expert at anything usually requires going through some steps again and again. Along the way we gain understanding.

Think back to your "aha!" moments, those times when you've suddenly had a big insight. Often they arrive after you've mulled over the same problem many times. Recall what it's like to return to one of your favorite books or movies. Chances are you discover things you never noticed were there.

The same thing applies when you're trying to change. Often you need to try things several times before you understand their value.

That's why we're going to take time this week to revisit some earlier territory. We've selected four activities from previous chapters that are well worth repeating.

ACTIVITY ALERT

Four Easy Activities

In addition to what you're doing to meet the goals you've set for yourself, we'd like you to do four simple activities. You can do them in any order. If you're worried about finding the time, sit down with your calendar and schedule each activity in advance. We've provided a form for you to use.

1. Hit the One-Half Mile Mark (Again)

In week 6, we asked you to map a one-half mile (.8 km) course in your neighborhood, walk it at a brisk pace, and see how long it took. We're going to ask you to do the same thing again. Return to your one-half mile (.8 km) route and walk it again, timing yourself. This time, compare how you feel walking with the way you felt the first time. Is it easier? Do you feel more confident? Did you complete the walk in less time? Did you feel less tired? If so, chances are you've already improved your fitness. (If you haven't made noticeable improvement, check "Troubleshooting" on page 82 for some tips.)

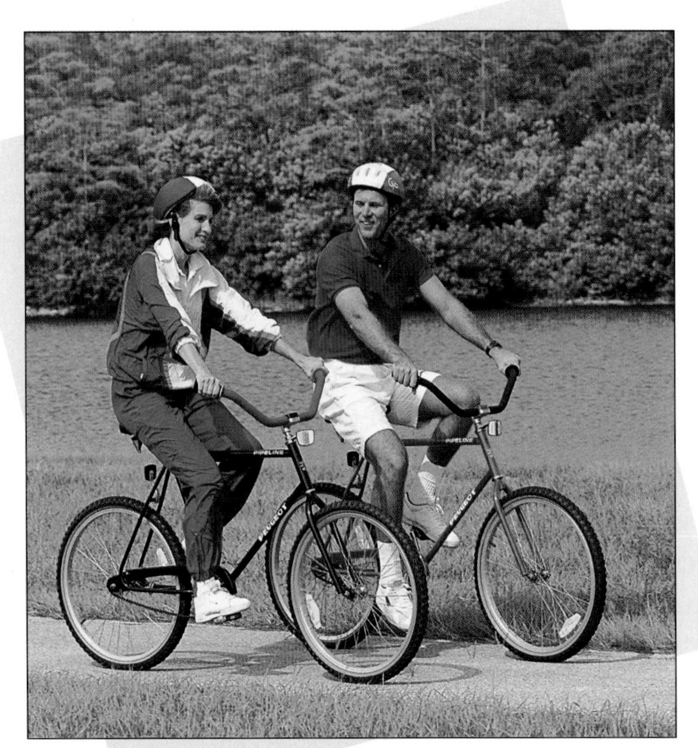

How about taking a bike ride with a friend?

2. Walk, Don't Drive

This one's easy: go shopping. Instead of circling the blocks or cruising the parking lot to find the nearest parking place, park your car at a distance and walk briskly to the store. (If you don't drive, get off the bus or subway at least one stop before the shopping area and walk.) While you're walking, look around and try to find something you hadn't noticed before—a new shop window, a particularly beautiful tree, even an interesting crack in the sidewalk. Add up the extra time you spend walking.

3. Find Some Company

At least once this week, turn a few minutes with a friend, family member, or coworker into an opportunity for activity. Suggest a walk in a nearby park or shopping mall. Plan a walk-and-talk business meeting. If you're feeling ambitious, and the weather is good, how about a spin on a bike? (Don't forget to wear a helmet!)

4. Watch TV

This may be the easiest of all: Watch TV. That's right—set aside an evening to watch a few of your favorite programs. Here's the catch: instead of vegging out during those long commercial breaks, walk around the house (or the block), dance to some music, or do some serious cleaning—anything that qualifies as moderate-intensity activity. Add up the extra minutes you spend being active.

FOUR SUREFIRE WAYS TO STAY ACTIVE

1. Measure your success.

Revisit the fitness tests you did in week 6. Measure your resting heart rate. Then do the walking test on page 49 again, and compare your previous scores and your new scores here.

	Previous	Date	Current	Date
Resting heart rate (beats per minute)				
Route completed time (minutes:seconds)				
Heart rate at route end (beats per minute)				

Chances are that if you have been staying active, you'll see a drop in your resting heart rate, time to complete your walking test, or your ending heart rate.

2. Walk, don't drive.

Where did you walk instead of drive?

____

(continued)

(continued)

Notice anything new?

____

3. Find some company.

Who joined you this week in activity?

____

What did you do together?

____

4. Watch TV.

How many minutes of activity did you accumulate during your favorite TV program?

____

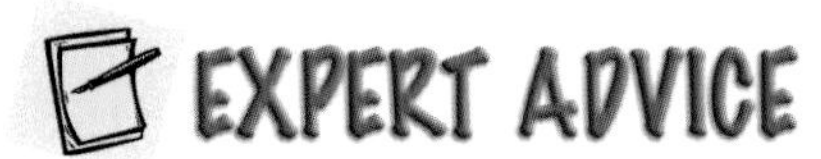

Troubleshooting: Getting Nowhere Fast?

Feeling frustrated by your progress or lack thereof? Is it still as hard as ever for you to push yourself through the paces? That means it's time for a little problem solving.

First, be honest with yourself. Have you been doing 30 minutes of moderate-intensity activity for several weeks? If not, you may need to work on being more consistent. Consistency is the key to building fitness.

If you have met your goal of 30 minutes most days of the week for several weeks, then it's time to check your pace. You may need to pick up the intensity a little to increase your fitness level. Don't go gangbusters. Simply try to increase your pace a little each week. Use a watch to record your time, if that helps, or monitor how winded you feel at the end of your activity. Push yourself a little harder each time and it won't be long before you see a difference. We guarantee it.

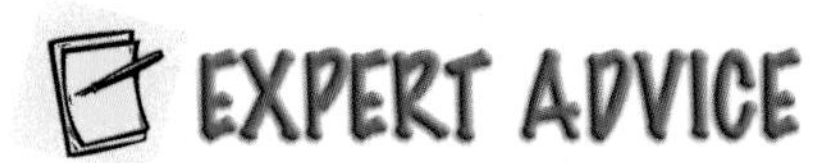

Stretching Exercises

Looking for a few simple stretching exercises you can do when you first wake up or between TV commercials? Try these four easy-to-do stretches:

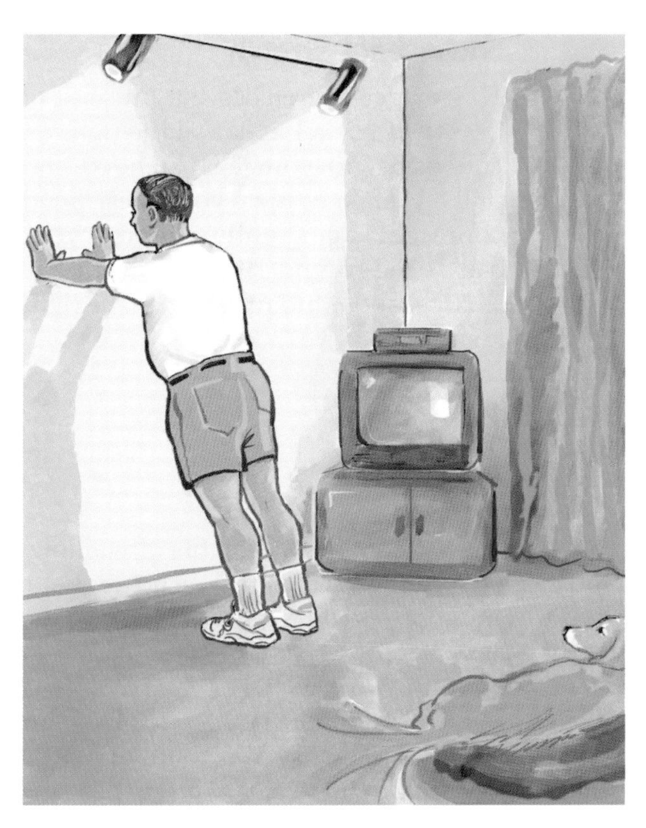

Achilles tendon and calf stretch

This exercise stretches the heel cord and the back of the lower leg. Stand two or three feet from a wall or tree with both toes pointed forward as you lean toward the wall, partly supporting yourself with your hands. Keep the heels flat to stretch the calf. Hold 10 to 20 seconds, and repeat.

Seated hamstring stretch

This exercise stretches the muscles of the back of the thigh. From a seated position with legs very slightly bent at the knees and hands on thighs, bend over slowly, reaching toward your toes. Keep your head and back straight as you move into the stretch. Hold 10 to 20 seconds, and repeat.

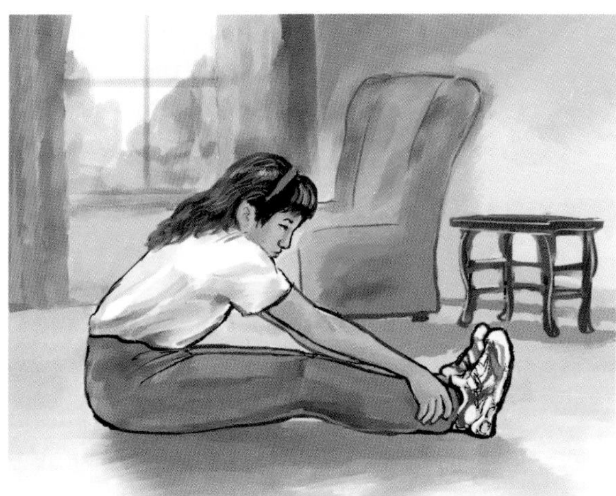

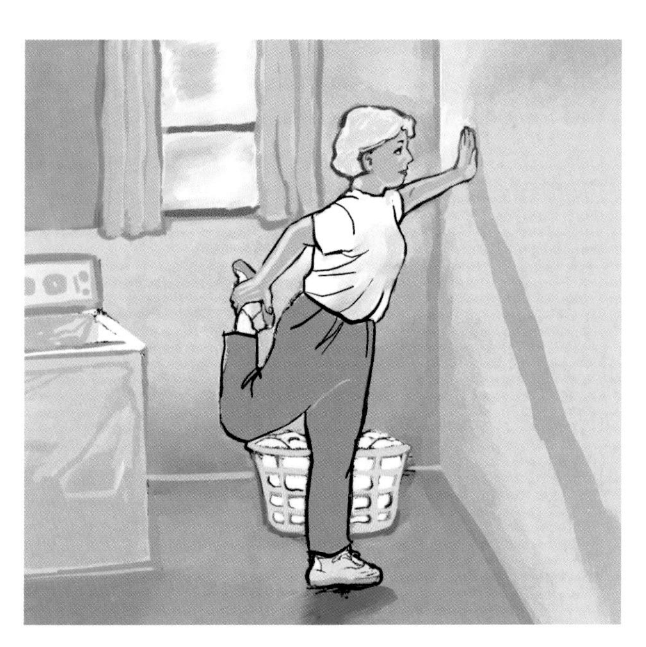

Quadriceps stretch

This exercise is to stretch the muscles of the front of the thigh. Place your left hand against a wall or tree for balance, then grab your right ankle with your right hand and pull it up and back toward your buttocks until you can feel a stretch on the front of your right thigh. Keep your back straight and your right knee pointing toward the ground. The standing leg should have a slightly bent knee. Hold the stretch for 10 to 20 seconds, then repeat with the left leg.

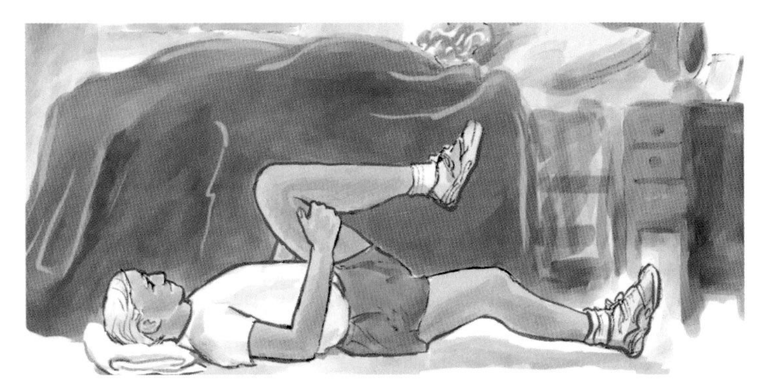

Lower back stretch

This exercise stretches the muscles of the lower back. Lie flat on the floor on your back with your legs extended, and pull the left knee up to your chest. Bend your right knee slightly and press your back to the ground. Hold the position 10 to 20 seconds, and repeat with the right knee.

UP CLOSE & PERSONAL

No matter how often he reminded himself about the benefits of walking, Will still found it boring. Worse yet, it felt like a waste of time he might be using for something more worthwhile. So despite his best intentions, he often skipped the walk. Over time, he began to fall short of his goal to walk at least five nights a week after dinner.

Then for Christmas his wife gave him a Walkman-style tape player and tapes of three of his favorite pieces of music. The first time out, he was so caught up in the music that he walked an extra three blocks just to hear the end of the piece. As a reward for meeting his goals each month, he began to treat himself to a new tape. It was a great way to become physically active and build his music collection.

NEED A BOOST?

Having a hard time meeting your goals? Never fear. Everyone encounters obstacles now and then. Here are some tips that can help you keep on track:

- Look back over the material in the previous week or two to find ideas or strategies to help you meet your activity goals.
- Post a list of the benefits you want to get from physical activity in a conspicuous place, such as the refrigerator, the TV, or your car dashboard.
- Visualize yourself as an active person. Think about how you'll spend your time and how you'll feel. Imagine the benefits you'll gain from increasing your activity.
- Ask someone close to you to help you problem solve the issues that are holding you back.
- Remember, becoming active for life is a process—it's not something you can expect to do overnight. Be patient. Set small goals.
- Give yourself a break. If you can't keep up, take the pace a little slower. Spend two weeks on a chapter.
- Keep track of your plans, goals, and activities. Keeping an activity log is a powerful motivator.
- Resolve to put activity high on your list of priorities. If you're not convinced, look back over the benefits of an active life that mean the most to you.

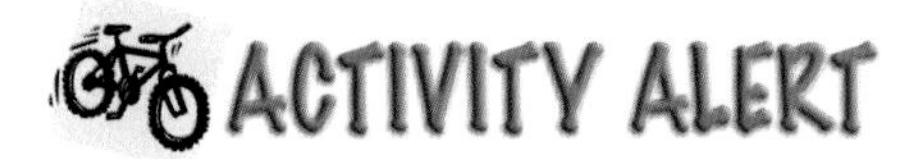

Whaddya Know?

That's right—it's pop quiz time. Don't worry, we're not handing out grades. Because we're almost halfway through, we thought it might be a good time to revisit a few key points. We're trying to strengthen the foundation here. What better way than testing your mastery with a few multiple choice questions?

1. As you increase your activity, your resting heart rate will
   a. increase
   b. decrease
   c. remain the same
2. Moderate-intensity activities are equivalent to
   a. brisk walking
   b. raking
   c. mopping floors
   d. bicycling at 10 miles (16 km) per hour
   e. all of the above
3. Which of the following burns the fewest calories in an hour?
   a. walking
   b. climbing stairs
   c. shopping
   d. watching TV
   e. gardening
4. The factors that determine the number of calories you burn in physical activity are
   a. duration
   b. frequency
   c. body weight
   d. intensity
   e. all of the above
5. Health experts now recommend accumulating 30 minutes of at least moderate-intensity activity
   a. once a week
   b. three times a week
   c. most days of the week
   d. every other day
6. The average television commercial break between shows lasts
   a. 30 seconds
   b. one minute
   c. one and one-half minutes
   d. two minutes or more

1. b; 2. e; 3. d; 4. e; 5. c; 6. d

Chapter Checklist

Before you move on to the next week's activities, make sure you

- Completed the four simple activities on pages 80-81
- Filled in the Four Surefire Ways to Stay Active form
- Practiced a few stretching exercises
- Tested your knowledge with the pop quiz on page 85

If you scored 100 percent on the multiple choice quiz, good for you. Treat yourself to something special. If you've met your short-term goals for the last couple weeks, it's also time for a reward. In the coming week, we'll look at why rewarding yourself is important when it comes to making a lifelong change.

WEEK **ELEVEN**

Rewarding Yourself

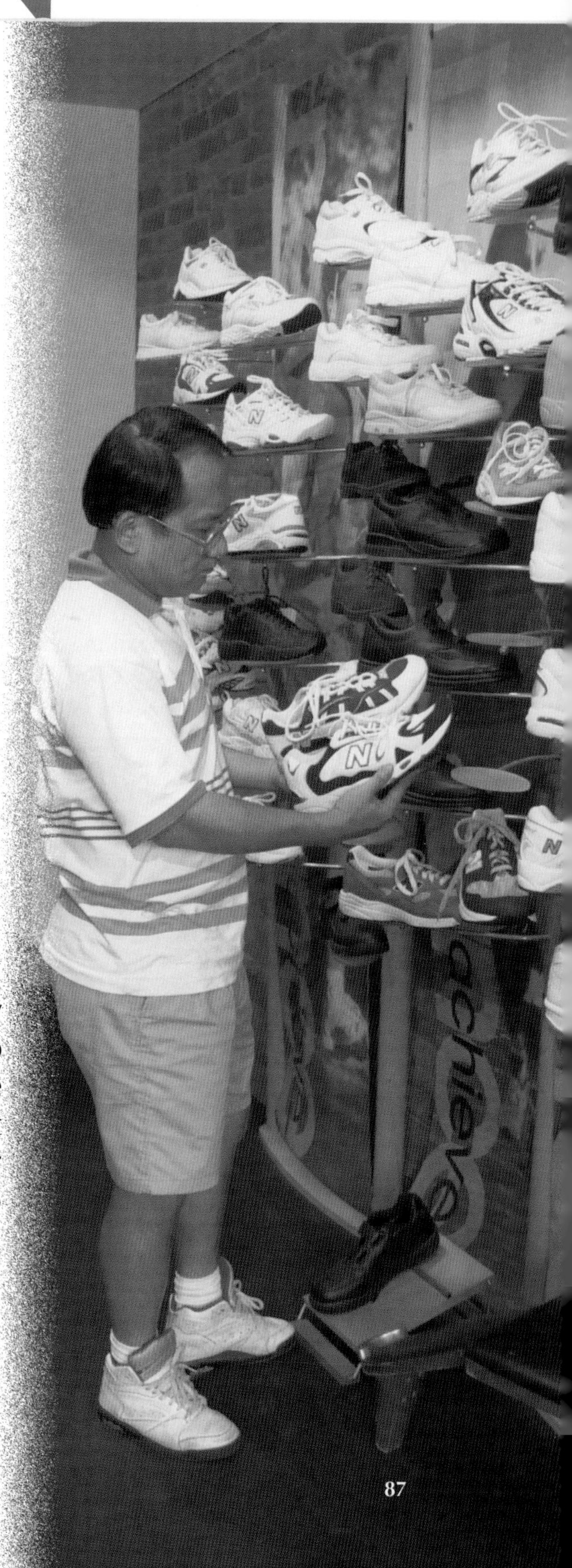

In This Chapter

- Identifying rewards that will keep you motivated
- Writing down positive messages
- Linking goals to specific rewards

If you've ever trained a puppy, you know how important small rewards can be. Most of us are no different. We reach further and achieve more when we know there's a reward waiting for us at the end of the line. The feeling of satisfaction after finishing a race may be its own reward, but it's also nice to get that T-shirt at the finish line.

Value of Rewards

The same goes for meeting your particular short- and long-term goals. There's an intrinsic reward that comes from feeling confident and in control, as well as healthy and energetic. That's important, but sometimes it helps to have planned an extrinsic reward, too—something tangible like a special book, theater tickets, a fancy dinner out, even a vacation—for when you attain your goal.

OK, and what if you haven't? What if you still have a way to go to meet your goal? Rewards can help focus your efforts and boost your motivation. Rewards are especially important as a way to get you over the rough patches when you're feeling discouraged or frustrated—and they happen to everyone.

UP CLOSE & PERSONAL

Louis was doing fine, working out regularly and keeping his weight and cholesterol down. Then his company transferred him to a new location. Suddenly he couldn't find time to get to the gym, and within a few months his cholesterol was up and his waistline was expanding.

Louis decided to work on the problem in small steps. He set out a program of specific goals with rewards over a six-month period. The first month's goal was to walk 10 minutes a day before breakfast and to increase his walking time each week by 10 minutes until he was up to an hour, five days a week. At the end of six months, he decided he would arrange for a vacation at the beach for the whole family.

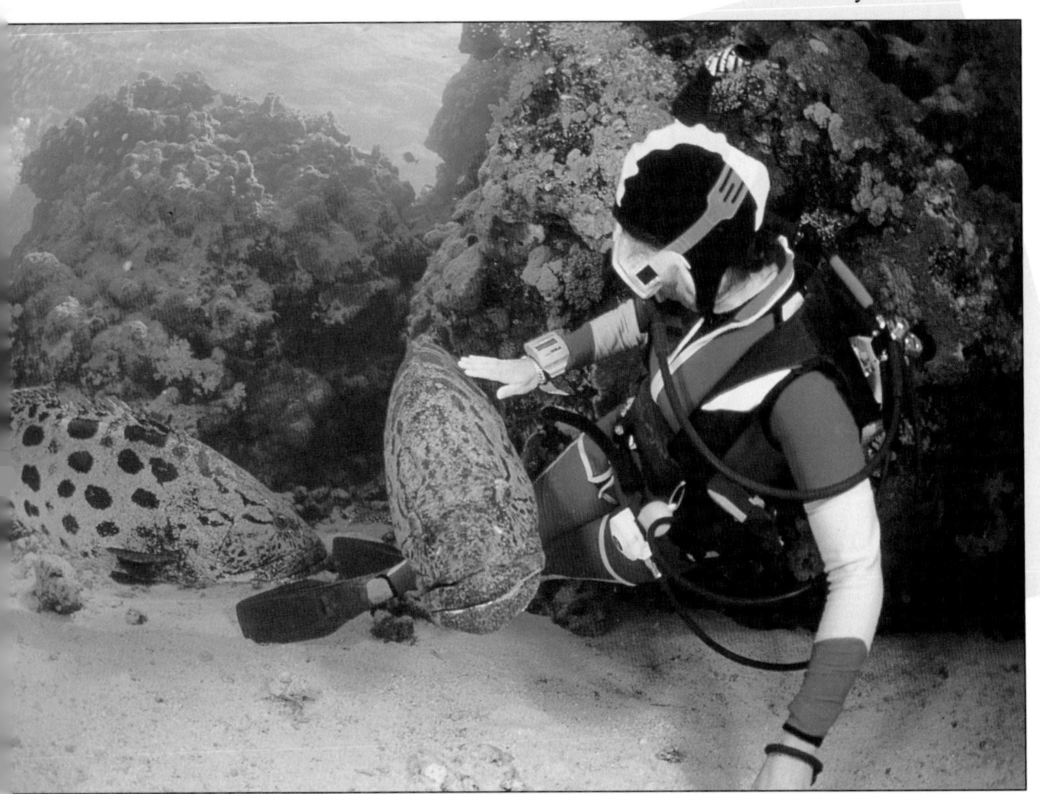

How can you reward yourself for a job well done?

Perhaps the smartest thing Louis did was tell his wife and family about his goal and the reward he'd promised himself when he reached it. His wife began to call him at work just before lunchtime to encourage him. At home his kids cheered him on. Every week he gave himself a small reward: a video he wanted to see or a new CD or music tape. Halfway through the six-month period, he began to feel discouraged because he wasn't losing weight as quickly as he'd hoped. He reminded himself that it was going to be a slow process, but every extra calorie expended would help.

He also found another terrific motivator. He and his wife decided that they would do something they'd always wanted—go scuba diving on their vacation. As they planned the trip, Louis got increasingly motivated to reach his goal. He wanted to have enough energy to enjoy diving. Most of all, he wanted to make sure he earned the reward of a special vacation. By the fourth month, he and his wife were both walking half an hour in the morning or in the evening, and Louis had added another 30 minutes by taking short 10-minute walks throughout the day.

EXPERT ADVICE

Zen of Activity

One important reward of an active lifestyle, as you know, is improved health and increased energy. If you're beginning to feel a little more fit now than before you increased your activity—with energy to spare when you need it to run for the bus or climb a steep set of stairs—chances are good you're already getting the health benefits of activity.

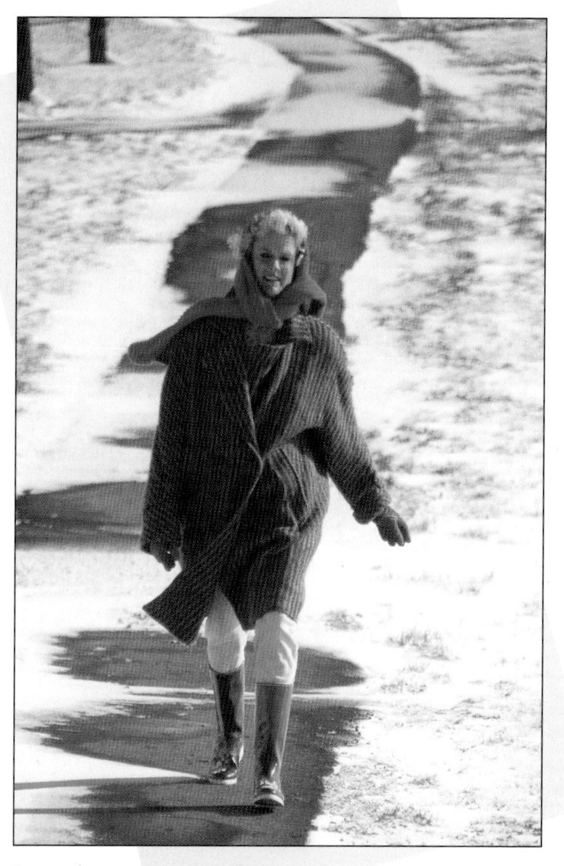

Savor the experience of physical activity!

However, don't ignore the here-and-now benefits that come with enjoying what you're doing. Physical activity should be fun. Moving, feeling your heart kick up, seeing the world around you, improving your self-confidence—all are important pleasures. The next time you engage in physical activity, whether it's walking, dancing, bicycling, or swimming, take a few minutes to savor the experience. Enjoy the sights, sounds, and smells you encounter along the way. Feel your arms and legs moving. Be aware of your heart beating. After you're through with the activity, take in a deep breath and let it out slowly.

It feels great to be active.

Creative Rewards

You would think rewarding ourselves would be easy. Often it's not. We're used to congratulating and encouraging our kids or spouses or loved ones, but most of us don't take time to congratulate ourselves.

Stumped for ideas on how to reward yourself? Here are a few of the special treats that worked well for Project *Active* participants:

Massage

Cool new running shoes

Theater or sports tickets

Bottle of wine

New hairdo

Bracelet

New watch

Bubble bath

New workout clothes

New portable audiotape or CD player

Dance class

Night out for dancing

New magazine or newsletter subscription

Flying a kite with friends or family

New pair of comfortable work shoes

Biking vacation

Manicure or facial

Night at a bed-and-breakfast

Fresh flowers

Small piece of chocolate

Visit with friends

Trip to a local museum

Movie

Dinner at your favorite restaurant

New CD or audiotape

New bike

New walking shoes

New blouse or shirt

Alone time for yourself

? DID YOU KNOW?

In our Project *Active* program and in our studies at Brown University, we measured the strategies that people used to meet their goals. People who increased their use of rewards were far more likely to remain active over time than those who didn't give themselves more rewards. Remember, the goal of this program is to help you make physical activity a lifelong habit.

ACTIVITY ALERT

Identifying Rewards

It's time to reward yourself for all the good work you're doing or plan to do. Think about your specific goals, both short and long term. Now make a list of a few ways you can reward yourself for achieving your short-term goals. (If your goal is to lose weight, of course, a fudge sundae may not be the best reward. Choose a reward that helps you move toward your goal, not away from it!)

____

____

____

____

Now think big. Write down ideas for rewards that might help spur you on to reaching your long-term goal.

____

____

____

____

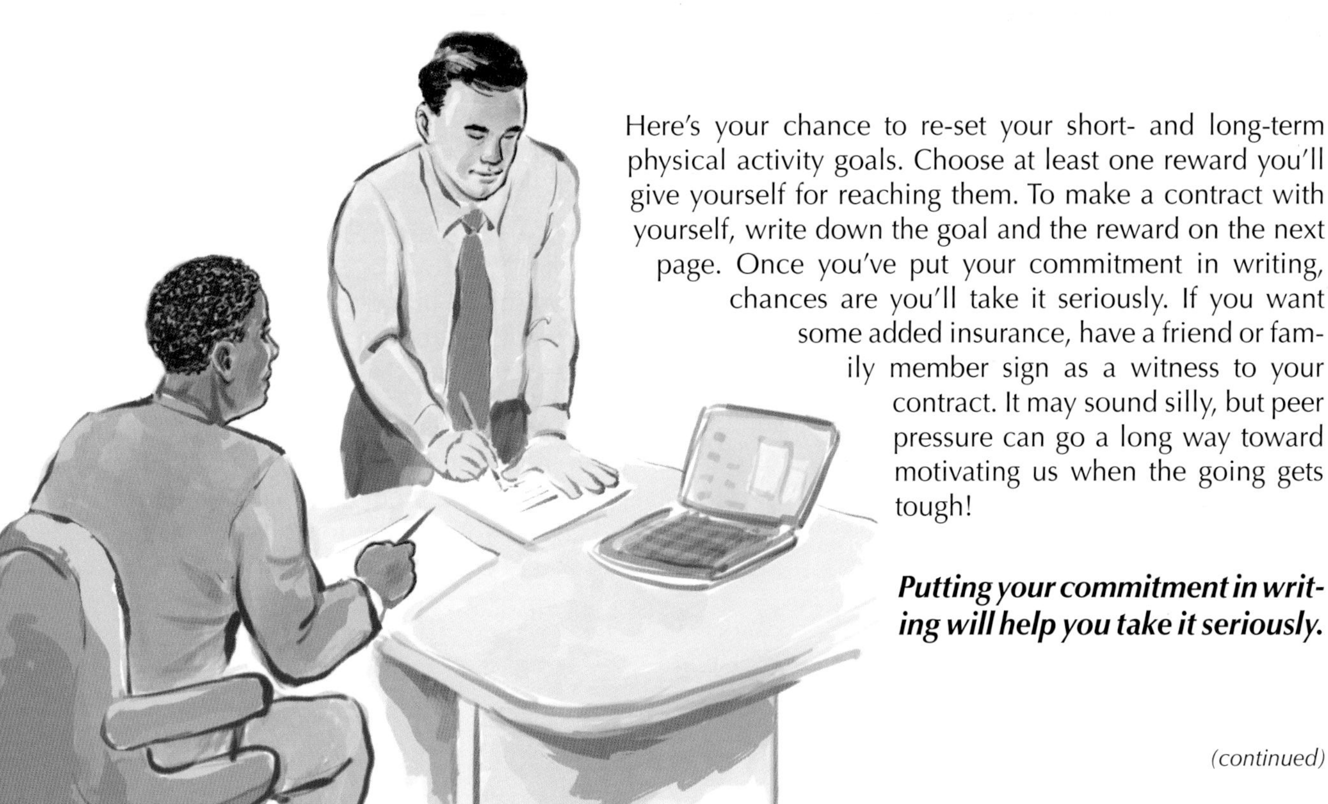

Here's your chance to re-set your short- and long-term physical activity goals. Choose at least one reward you'll give yourself for reaching them. To make a contract with yourself, write down the goal and the reward on the next page. Once you've put your commitment in writing, chances are you'll take it seriously. If you want some added insurance, have a friend or family member sign as a witness to your contract. It may sound silly, but peer pressure can go a long way toward motivating us when the going gets tough!

Putting your commitment in writing will help you take it seriously.

(continued)

(continued)

MY CONTRACT

When I meet my short-term goal, which is

____

I will reward myself with

____

When I reach my long-term goal, which is

____

I will reward myself with

____

ACTIVITY ALERT

Pat Yourself on the Back

The messages we give ourselves can have a big impact on what we achieve. If the messages are negative, such as "I'm no good at sticking with a plan" or "I'm always too tired at the end of the day to do anything," it's easy to get discouraged. However, if you encourage yourself with positive messages, such as "All I need is 10 minutes to relax, then I'm ready for anything" or "I can do anything if I put my heart into it," chances are you'll succeed.

Take a few minutes now to think of some positive things to say to yourself about being physically active. Some examples might be the following:

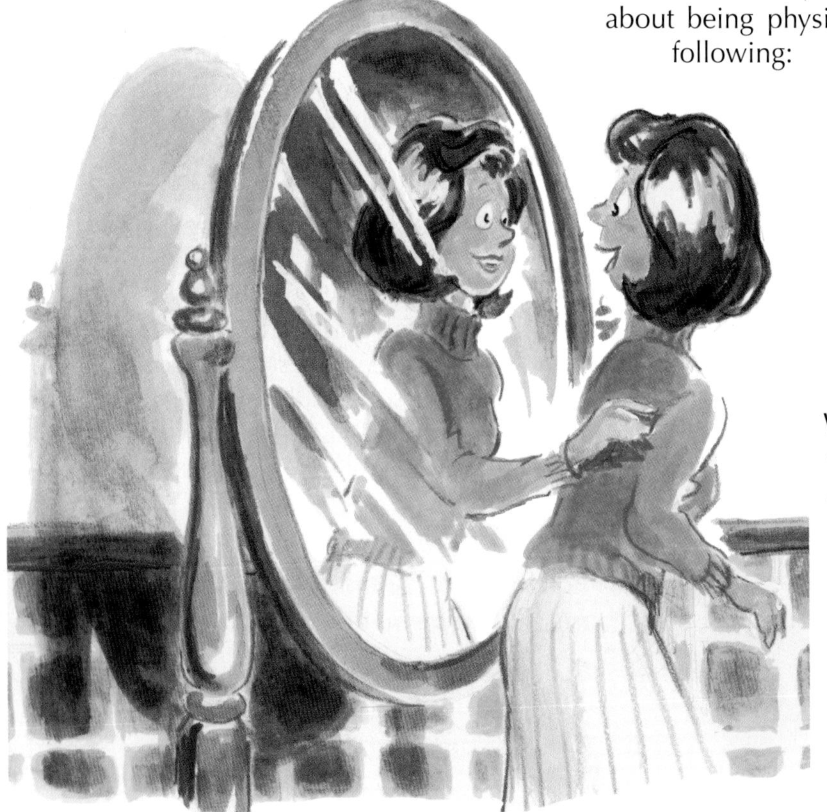

- "It may be hard for me to get going sometimes, but once I get over that first hurdle, there's no stopping me."
- "Just getting up and moving makes me feel better."
- "I've solved bigger problems. I can figure out where to find another 10 minutes for activity."

Write down at least two messages that will work to inspire and encourage you. (You may also want to write them on a piece of paper you keep in your wallet for those moments when you need a little push.)

____

____

DID YOU KNOW?

In treating diabetes, a lot of attention is focused on proper dietary practices. Diet is important, but new data from The Cooper Institute[10] show that physical activity and fitness are also extremely important for reducing risk of premature death in men with diabetes. We found that men who had diabetes and were unfit were *twice* as likely to die prematurely as fit men with diabetes. This association was present even when considering other common risk factors such as high blood pressure, high blood cholesterol, smoking, obesity, family history of heart disease, and alcohol intake. We know that being physically active is important for otherwise healthy people. This study shows that even people who have a difficult medical condition can benefit as well. A new study from Harvard School of Public Health suggests that moderate and vigorous physical activity may reduce the risk of getting type 2 diabetes in women.[11] Just a few more rewards for being active!

UP CLOSE & PERSONAL

Mariel had gone through a tough year. She'd lost her job as a receptionist when the company moved, and it had taken her almost two months to find another job. A single mom with two small kids, she had to watch every penny. With the stress of being unemployed, she stopped going out for walks and began eating junk food. Within a month she had gained six pounds. Worse than that, she began to think of herself as a failure in almost everything she did.

Luckily, she knew herself well enough to know that wasn't true. To counter the negative message, she wrote a list of the things she was proud of accomplishing. Her list included "No matter how tired I feel, I can always find energy to play with the kids," and "Once I set a goal, I can reach it."

Those two insights helped her out of her rut. She immediately set a goal to take three brisk walks each day for the rest of the week. She also made plans to take the kids to the playground after school, where they could all be active together. When she finally found another job, one that paid more than her previous job, she rewarded herself and the kids with a day at a local amusement park.

Chapter Checklist

Before you move on to the next week's activities, make sure you

- Made a contract to reward yourself for meeting a short-term goal
- Made a contract to reward yourself for meeting a long-term goal
- Made a list of positive messages to encourage yourself

A specific reward will focus your commitment and help you over the rough patches. Along the way, it's important to talk positively to yourself. It will help you stay motivated to achieve your goals. But even rewards and positive thinking aren't guarantees. Most of us stumble and fall sometimes and have a tough time getting back on track. In the next week we'll look at how to make sure that a lapse doesn't lead to a relapse, or worse yet, a collapse.

WEEK **TWELVE**

Avoiding Pitfalls

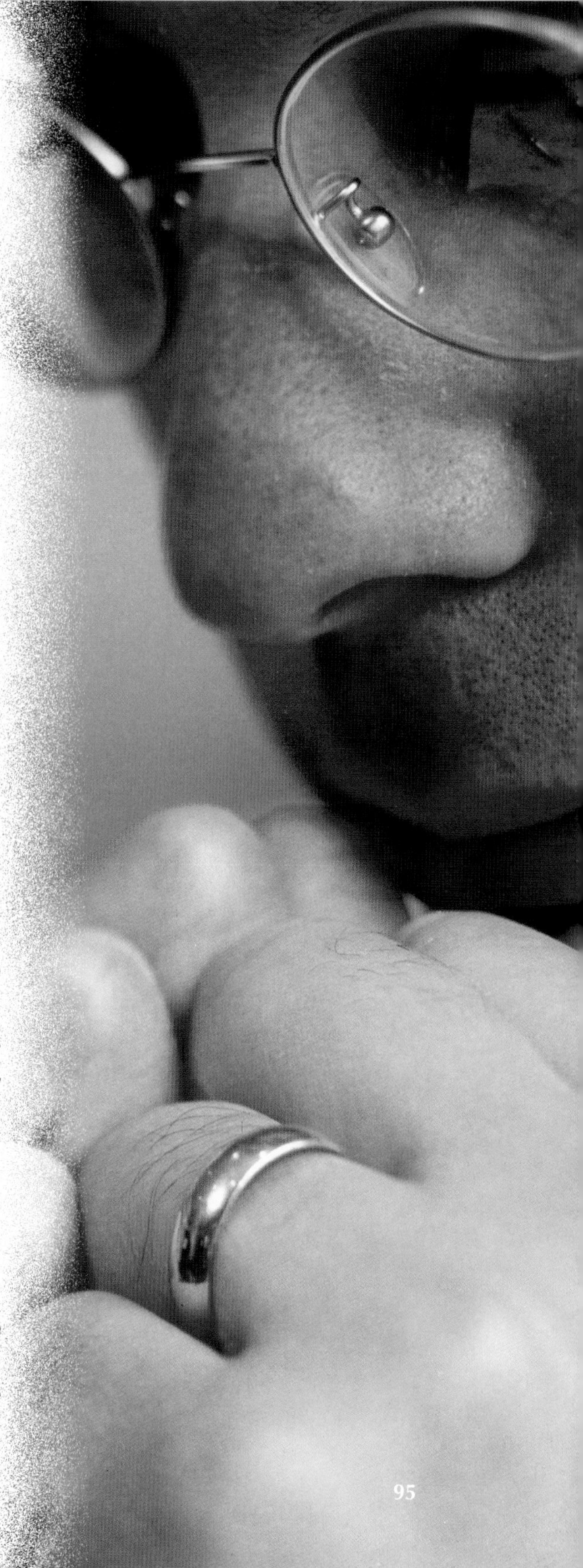

In This Chapter

- Recognizing the all-or-nothing trap
- Identifying pitfalls that can trip you up
- Planning for high-risk situations

We've said it before, but it's worth repeating: no matter how good your intentions are, at certain points along the way you're likely to falter. Maybe you're doing fine until the holidays hit and your schedule goes awry. Maybe you have a hectic stretch at work or a rocky period in a relationship. Perhaps you injured yourself or came down with the flu. Whatever the reason, there are times when it's tough to stick to your plan for physical activity. That's unavoidable. What you can avoid is letting a brief lapse turn into a full-fledged collapse. In this chapter we'll look at strategies to deal with the rough times.

EXPERT ADVICE

All-or-Nothing Trap

One of the first mistakes people make when they fall short of their goal is to think, "That's it, I've blown it. I'll never make this work. Maybe I'm just destined to be a couch potato."

Don't believe it. A one-time slip doesn't mean you're a failure. It doesn't mean you're fated to be sedentary. That's the all-or-nothing trap, and plenty of people with the best intentions have fallen into it. People mistakenly think, "Either I stick to my plan and meet my goal, or I'm a failure."

The fact is, all-or-nothing thinking is taking the easy way out. It's a fancy way of quitting. Maybe you've missed a day or two of activity. Maybe you've blown a whole week. Maybe you've been sick, injured yourself, or run into some family trouble, and you've been out of commission for a month or more. The important point is to understand it for what it is: a *lapse*. Sure you've fallen a step behind, but your hard work is not lost. Remind yourself of all you've learned and how far you've come since you started. Look back through this book if you need proof that you've made progress. With a little effort you can take two steps forward and keep up the progress you've been making.

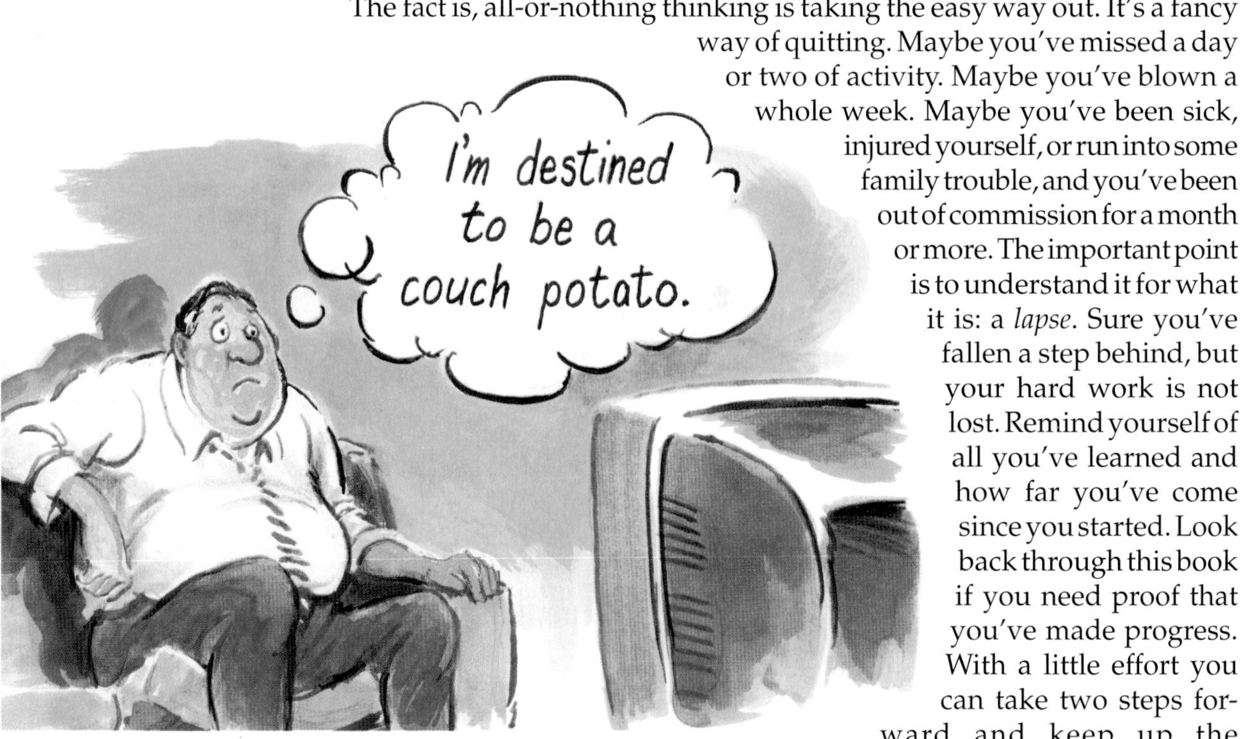

One thing you don't want to do is give up.

The key to recovering from a lapse is to act fast and get active immediately. Here's what to do:

Be honest. Admit to yourself that you've hit a snag. Figure out exactly how long you've lapsed and think about what knocked you off track.

Turn to your support troops. If you've gotten support and encouragement from friends or loved ones, now is the time to turn to them for another pep talk. Again, be honest. No one likes to admit that they've faltered, but by telling someone, you may be able to enlist help to get out of the rut and back on track.

Start self-monitoring immediately. Look back at the Personal Time Study form on pages 11-12. If your schedule has changed significantly since you last filled it in, you may want to update your Personal Time Study. Either way, the point is to identify opportunities to fit in activity. Write them down on your calendar.

Set new goals. This is a good time to look back at your current plan and goals. Think about ways you might revise them to make them work better for you. To renew your motivation, look for ways to incorporate activities you enjoy. If you've been sick or injured, don't let it be an excuse to stop permanently. Set a date when you will start again. You may need to work up slowly to the level you were at before. That's fine. The important thing is to commit yourself to a goal of getting back into an active lifestyle. Give yourself a little time, and you'll regain all the lost ground.

Avoid negative messages. Remember those discouraging voices that sometimes speak up when things go wrong—the voices that say things such as "failure," "can't," or "never"? Now is the time to counter those negative messages with positive ones. Instead of saying, "I can't stick to my plan," remind yourself that you did fine for the first month, and come up with a plan for what you can do from now on.

Focus on your strengths. This is another way to accentuate the positive. Look back over the period when you were doing well. Think about the personal strengths you discovered. Maybe you learned that you like doing activities with other people. Perhaps you found that you achieve more if you have a specific plan and a schedule for meeting your goal. Like some participants in our program, you may have been surprised to discover that you enjoy certain activities, such as dancing or roller-blading. Enjoying activities is an important strength you can leverage. Once you've identified your personal strengths, think about ways to use them now to get yourself back in the game.

UP CLOSE & PERSONAL

Fran and her husband Eddie were into their eighth week of walking 30 minutes after dinner every weeknight. They'd rediscovered the pleasures of seeing the neighborhood and spending quiet time together. Fran had even begun to see an improvement in the mirror—something she was hoping for.

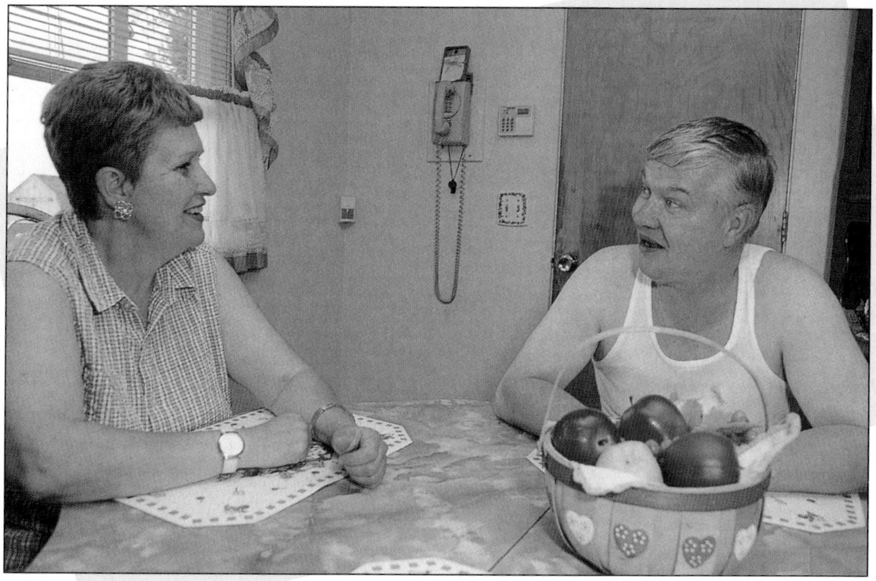

A spouse or friend can offer encouragement when pitfalls occur.

Then trouble struck. Lifting a heavy box at work, she wrenched her back so badly that by the next morning she could barely get out of bed. She spent a week recuperating at home, then another week going into work just half days. A month passed before the pain had subsided enough to allow her to walk any distance at all.

Eddie wanted to keep up the activity, but with

Fran injured he had to take on most of the household duties. He could see the frustration in Fran's face when she couldn't go out walking. He didn't want to hurt her feelings by leaving her alone in the house while he walked.

The upshot was that after going strong for two months, they did nothing for a whole month. A lapse was beginning to turn into a full-fledged collapse. The truth is, Fran was ready to give up completely. But Eddie reminded her how good both of them had felt and how much pleasure they'd gotten out of their walks. Also, he was sure walking would help Fran recover faster than if she wasn't active. One day he sat down with her and told her how important it was to him that the two of them get back on track. He asked how much she thought she could do. They revised their goals to begin with a 10-minute walk and set a date on the calendar to begin again. For an added incentive, Eddie picked up a brand new pair of walking shoes for Fran. Within a month they were back to walking 30 minutes every evening.

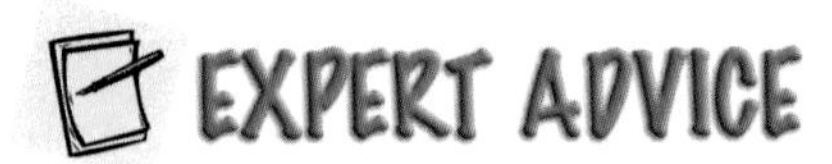

Trouble Ahead

Sometimes trouble comes out of nowhere—an injury, for example, or a family crisis. But more often, the potholes in the road to success are easy to anticipate. As long as you know what situations cause problems, you can avoid being ambushed by them. All it takes is recognizing trouble and preparing strategies to get through it. Here are three high-risk situations and simple tips on how to steer clear of a lapse:

Emotional Upsets

Minor or major crises, or simply a high level of everyday stress, can undermine your motivation. It's natural to think, "I'm too stressed to fit physical activity into my schedule right now." The solution is to remind yourself that being physically inactive isn't going to improve the situation. In fact, taking a few moments for yourself and doing something you enjoy could be a great way to counter stress.

Business Trips

As long as we have our familiar schedules and settings, we can usually stick to our plans. But when we find ourselves in a new setting and an unfamiliar schedule, it's easy to get distracted. That's why business trips and vacations are many people's downfall.

The solution is to plan how you will maintain your physical activity. If you have a favorite pair of shoes, be sure to pack them. If there are no places to go for a walk at your hotel or you don't feel safe, check out other options: local shopping malls, local parks with walking paths, even the airport. Usually the hotel staff can advise you about safe places to walk when you arrive. If the weather outside is frightful, you can always use hotel hallways and stairs to walk and climb. Many hotels have pools, so be sure to pack a swimsuit. Even if you're not a regular swimmer, taking a plunge can be a great way to unwind after a long trip or an intense business meeting.

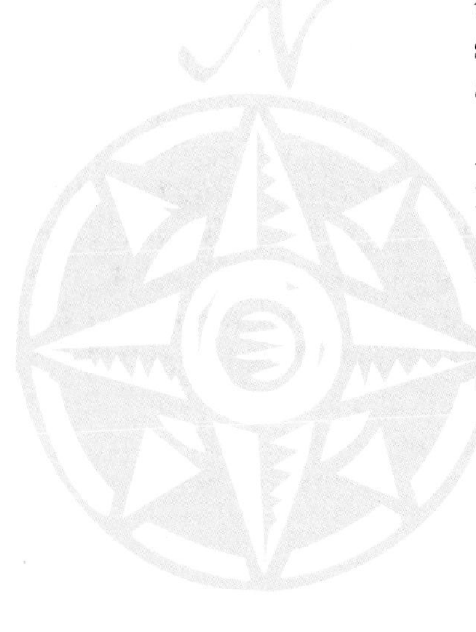

Vacations

Vacations also can throw your normal activity schedule awry. On top of that, many of us think of vacations as times to kick back and relax. That's fine, but activities you enjoy doing can be as relaxing as sitting on the beach.

Before you leave on vacation, make a list of physical activities you could do while away. Perhaps you want to stick with what you've been doing and just find the right time and place. However, vacations can offer many opportunities to try something new too, from hiking a trail in the Rockies to snorkeling in the Bahamas. You may even want to plan a vacation around an activity, such as cross-country skiing in Colorado or bicycling on Cape Cod. If you're visiting a large city, one of the best ways to see the sights is to get a map and do a walking tour. Also consider that you don't have to go anywhere. Sometimes the most rewarding vacations are spent at home catching up on things you need to do, such as cleaning the garage, painting the kitchen, or redoing the garden. Use these times to plan a family activity that everyone can do together. Try something new.

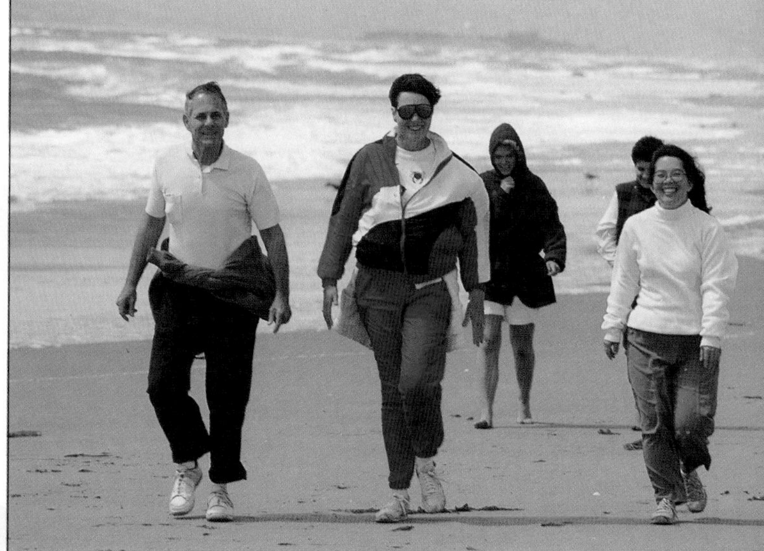

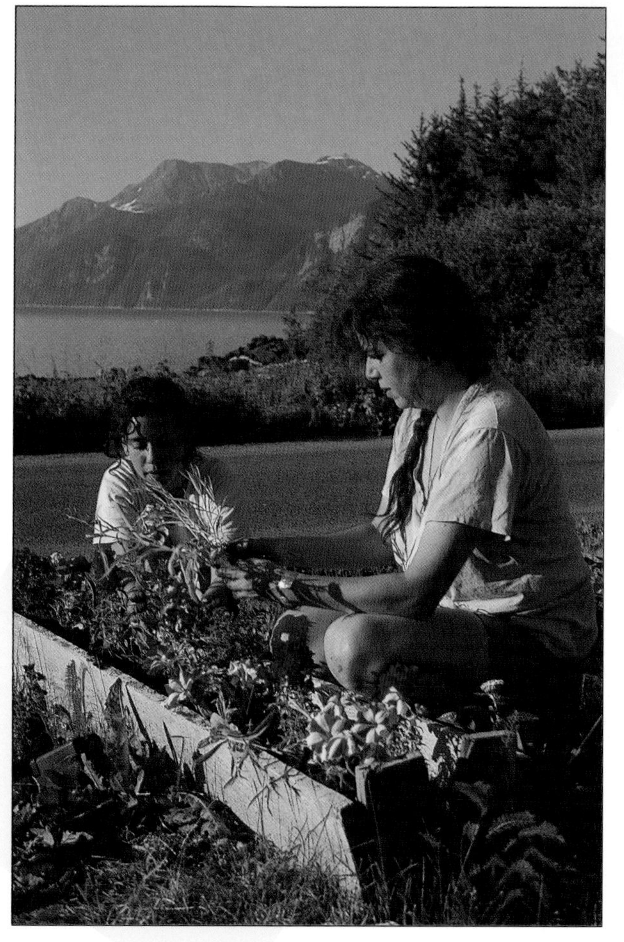

Even on business trips or vacations, you can find ways to be physically active.

? DID YOU KNOW?

Jumping on your bike for a spin around the neighborhood maybe a great way to reduce your risk for colon cancer. In Norway, researchers[12] found that as few as four hours of moderate cycling per week reduced the risk of colon cancer in women volunteers by almost 40 percent.

Worried about hurting yourself? First, be sure to wear a helmet, which reduces the risk of a serious head injury by about 85 percent. Second, check out local bike paths, which are likely to be the safest routes. Third, don't drink and ride. According to one recent study, 17 percent of cyclists admitted to the hospital for injuries were drunk at the time of the accident!

Your local bike shop can offer tips on equipment, local bike paths, and biking clubs.

If you don't own a bike, get the good old yellow pages out and look up bicycle rentals. Try it before you buy it! Used bicycles can be a real bargain. Often the police hold auctions to sell unclaimed bicycles. Of course, there's always the for sale ads. Bike shops are also a great resource for tips on how to select a bicycle that's a good fit for you; shops may offer assistance on where to ride and low-traffic routes.

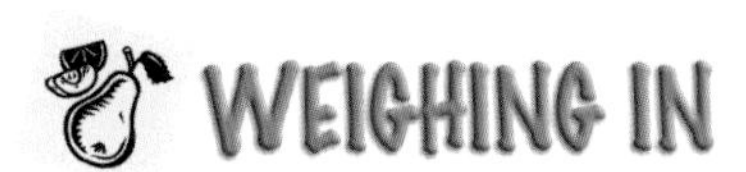

Holiday Weight Gain

Lots of special foods and no time to be active adds up to extra pounds during the holidays, or does it? A new study[13] shows that people averaged only a 1-pound (.45 kg) weight gain during the holidays instead of 5 pounds (2.26 kg) as was previously thought. The bad news is they didn't lose it over the rest of the year. Thus, many years of small holiday weight gains add up! Planning to stay active during the holidays is a good way to prevent weight gain and combat stress.

ACTIVITY ALERT

Planning for High-Risk Situations

There are plenty of obstacles out there. Here are the top six high-risk situations that cause people to falter. Check off those that are most likely to trip you up. Then go back and think about each situation. What does it feel like when you run into trouble? How could you plan to avoid trouble the next time it comes along? A few tips can help. First, define the problem by breaking it down into several manageable parts. Second, to avoid the problem, formulate a plan that is specific and achievable. Third, consider your strengths and resources, including friends, family, or resources in the community.

(continued)

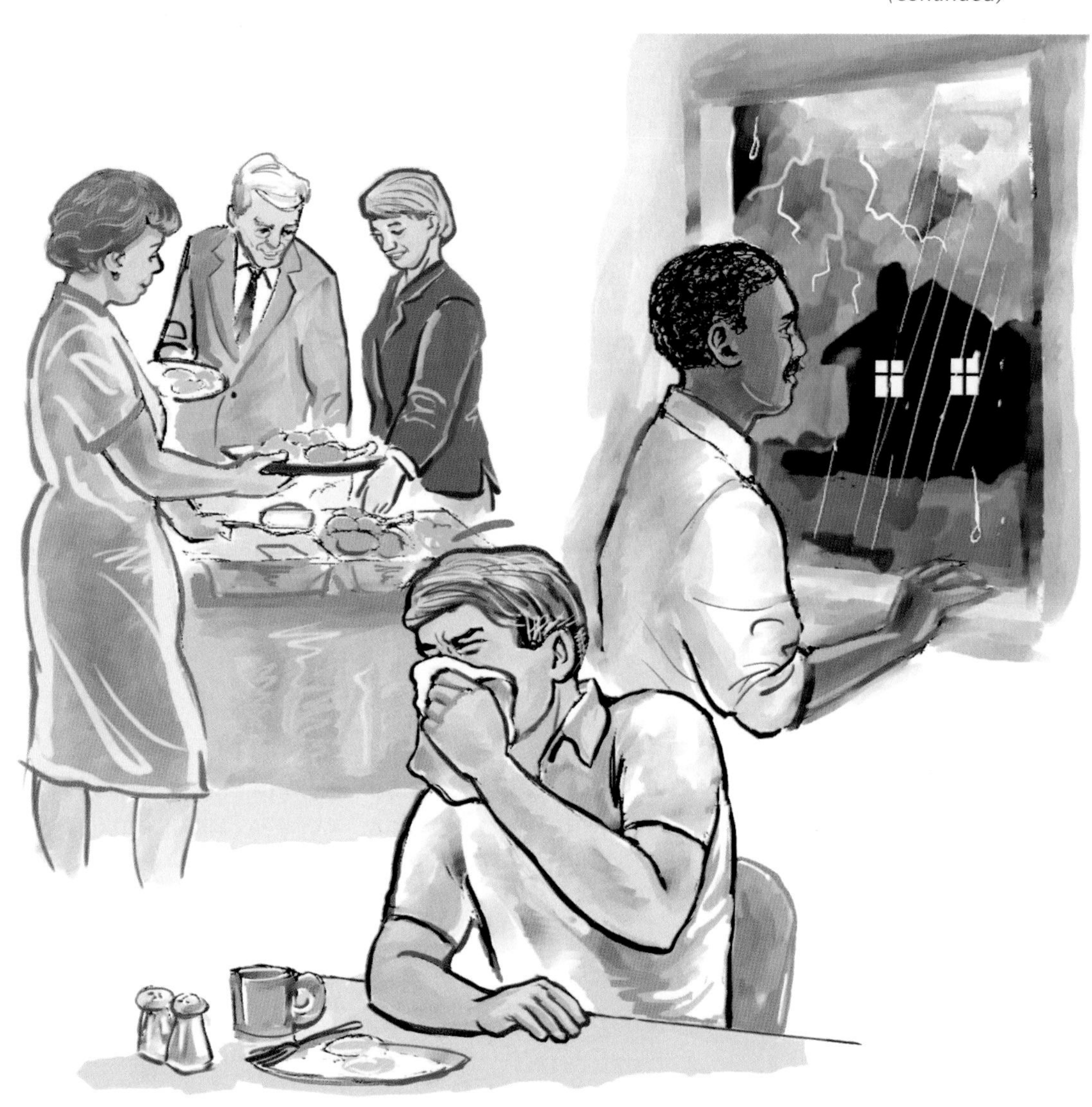

Can you relate to any of these high-risk situations?

(continued)

MY PLAN FOR HIGH-RISK SITUATIONS

❑ **Holiday madness**

It's December, and the entire family is coming to town for the holidays. Ho! Ho! Ho! You usually end up sitting around, eating too much, and getting almost no physical activity. The holidays have been your downfall before. What's the biggest problem you encounter?

____

____

____

What plan can you make now to stay on track and get more physical activity than you have in the past?

____

____

❑ **On the mend**

You've been sick all week with a rotten cold. The last two days you've spent in bed. At long last your throat is less scratchy and you're beginning to get your energy back. However, now that you've interrupted your regimen of activities, you're having a hard time getting yourself motivated again. What do you think about at a time like this?

____

____

____

How can you overcome your negative thinking to get back to your physical activity?

____

____

❑ **Crazy at work**

It's been a busy week at work, and there's no relief in sight. The deadlines just keep on coming. You've been working long days, and by the time you get home you're exhausted. Your plans for physical activity are beginning to totter. What are your thoughts and feelings?

____

____

____

Physical activity is a terrific antidote to stress. What plan can you make to fit it in, even during the busiest times?

____

____

❑ **Stormy weather**

It's too cold (hot, snowy, rainy, or humid) to go out and do anything. What are your thoughts at a time like this?

____

____

____

You can't buy the right weather, but you can buy the right gear or you can come up with alternatives that don't leave you out in the cold. What's your plan for dealing with foul weather?

____

____

❑ **Business travel**

You're traveling to an unfamiliar city for business. You've got some downtime when you could do something, but you're not sure what to do, or where. What are your thoughts and feelings at a time like this?

____

____

____

Many business travelers find they have more free time on the road than at home. What's your plan to use your free time for activity?

____

____

❑ **Good Samaritan**

You are unexpectedly called out of town to take care of a sick relative who has been hospitalized. The situation is uncertain and you don't know how long you'll be gone. What are your thoughts and feelings about sticking with your plan for physical activity?

____

____

____

Physical activity can help you stay in a positive frame of mind and cope. What positive messages and physical activities can you do to keep yourself going?

____

____

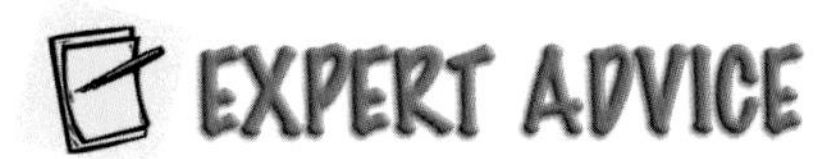

Avoiding Injuries

Nothing can sidetrack your efforts to be physically active faster than an injury. One leading cause of activity-related injuries is trying to do too much too fast. The best bet is to take a gradual approach. This helps strengthen muscles and stretch tendons slowly, reducing the chances of an injury. Knee injuries are one of the most common injuries. You can lower the odds of hurting yourself by strengthening the muscles above the knee, called the quadriceps, and by stretching and strengthening the muscles in the back of your upper leg, which are sometimes called hamstring muscles. For a few simple stretching exercises, check pages 82-84.

ACTIVITY ALERT

Preparing for High-Risk Situations

We've looked at how you can steer clear of high-risk situations by planning. The important thing is to spot trouble before it trips you up. Take a moment to list three of your high-risk situations. After each, list two or three things you can do to make sure a lapse doesn't turn into collapse.

High-risk situation 1

____

____

____

How to avoid trouble

____

____

____

High-risk situation 2

____

____

____

How to avoid trouble

____

____

____

High-risk situation 3

____

____

____

How to avoid trouble

____

____

____

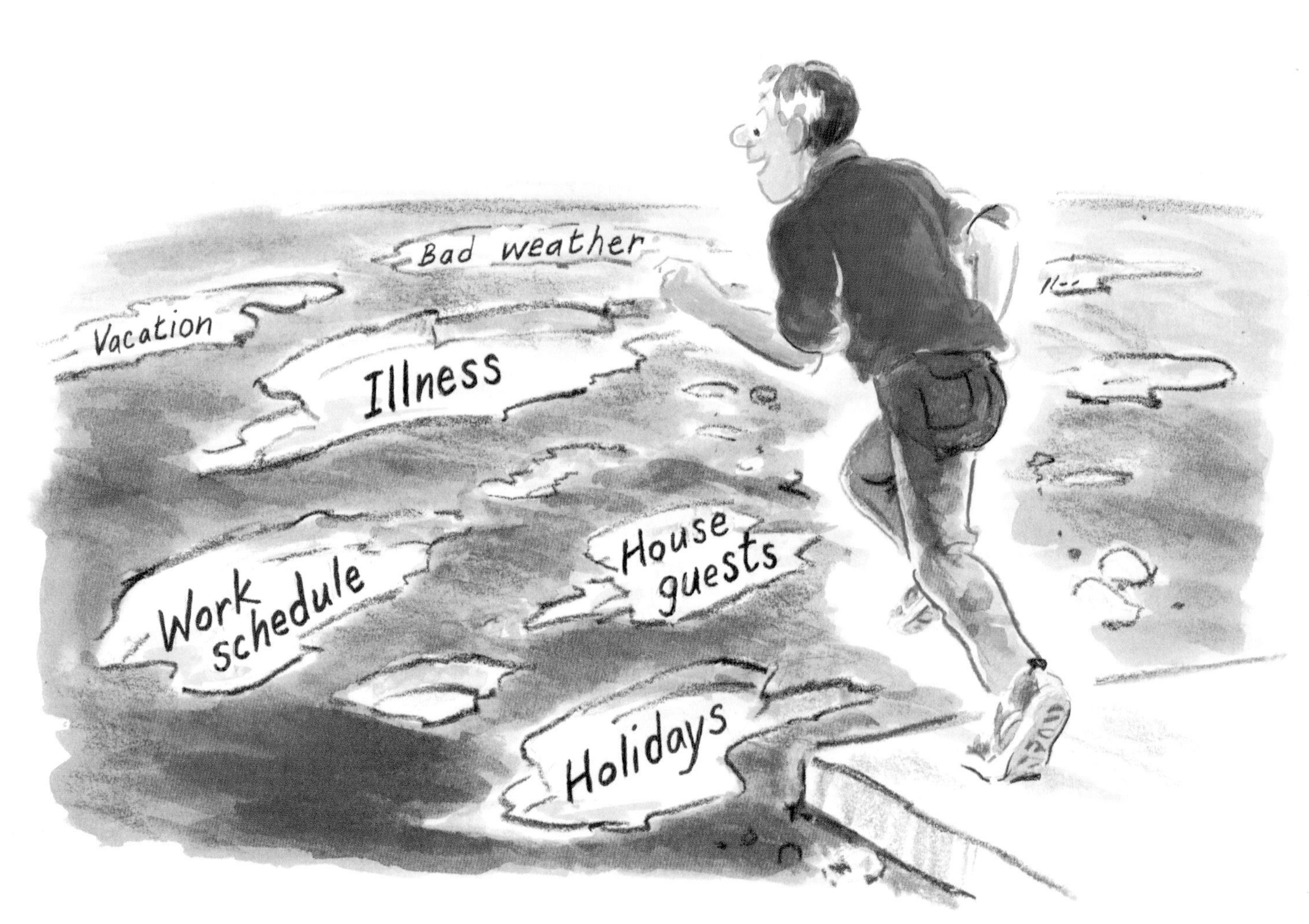

Which potholes do you need to plan for?

Chapter Checklist

Before you move on to the next week's activities, make sure you

- Learned to recognize all-or-nothing thinking
- Brainstormed about ways around high-risk situations
- Identified your high-risk situations

By now you've formulated some strategies to identify and sidestep problems before they knock you off track. One big challenge many people face in trying to change for the better is stress. Too much stress can rob you of energy and jeopardize your sense of well-being. Next week we'll look at a few ways to tame the wild beast of stress.

WEEK **THIRTEEN**

Defusing Stress

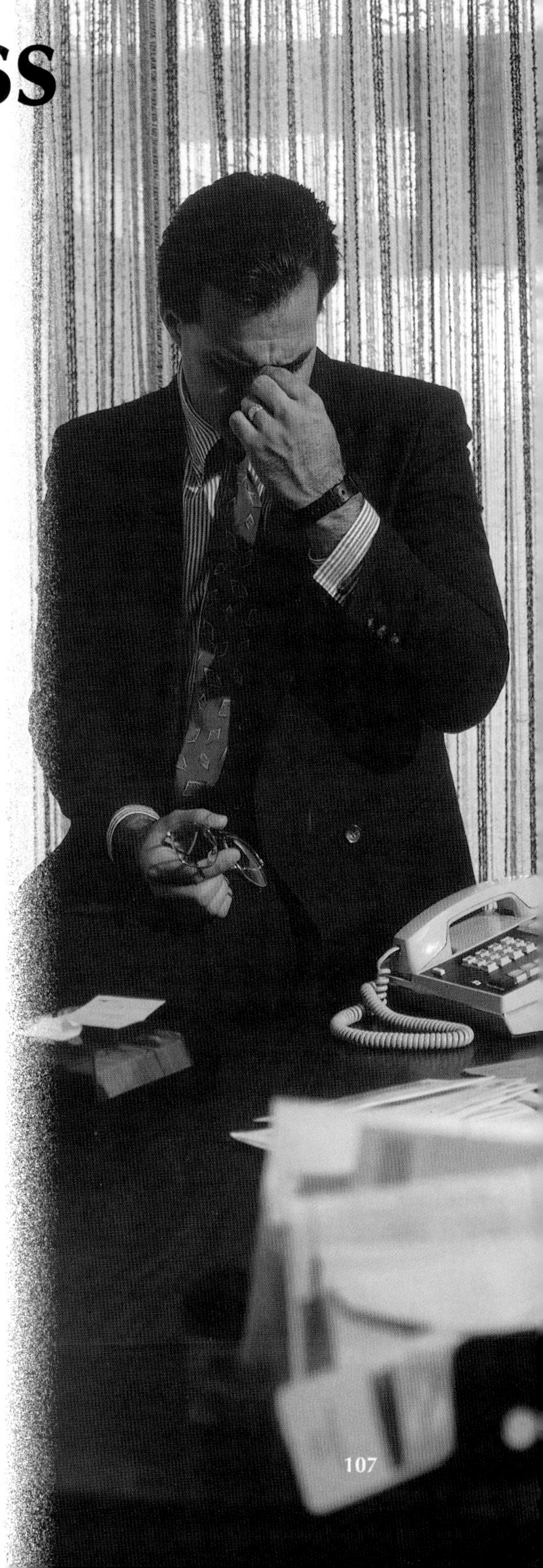

In This Chapter

- Learning about the risks of stress
- Identifying stressful situations
- Exploring four techniques to reduce stress
- Revisiting the stages of change

By now you are overcoming barriers to physical activity and have started planning for high-risk situations. But what if it is stress that trips you up? The stress of a new job, an illness, or a move can undermine your attempts to be physically active. This week you will identify stressors unique to you and learn ways to defuse that stress.

In week 3, we asked you to close this book, put it down, and take a walk. Now we're going to ask you to do something else you won't often see in a book about physical activity. Sit down and take a deep breath, filling your lungs with air from top to bottom. Draw the air in slowly, and just as slowly let it out. Then take another deep breath and let it out.

Go ahead and give it a try now.

Odds are good you feel calmer and more relaxed than before you paused to breathe. No matter how frazzled you may be feeling, taking a deep breath can help relieve tension. That's why breathing exercises are an important part of many stress-reduction techniques, including meditation and yoga.

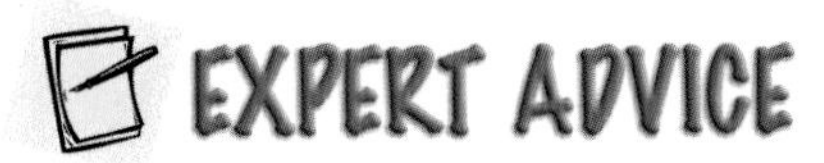

The Big Deal About Stress

Why worry about stress in a book about physical activity? There is one simple reason. High levels of stress can get in the way of making healthful changes in your life. It can wreak havoc with your motivation, which, as you have learned, is critical for your progression through the stages of change. People who are trying to give up smoking often falter during periods of high stress. That's when they feel they most need a cigarette. Stress can also get in your way when you're trying to stick to your goal of at least 30 minutes of physical activity most days of the week. When a period of high stress comes along, you may find yourself feeling distracted or discouraged—unless you find ways to let off some steam.

Stress comes in many forms. We usually associate it with negative events such as financial problems, marital difficulties, a bad period at work, or being sick. But stress can also occur during the good times, such as becoming engaged, having a child, buying a new car, or looking for your first home.

When something arises suddenly, then is over relatively quickly, such as having a flat tire or breaking a favorite pitcher, we typically experience *acute* stress. When something troubles us for days and weeks on end—an unhappy relationship, trouble with one of our kids, or an unpleasant boss—we typically experience *chronic* stress. Chronic stress causes the most damage in its effects on the body and mind.

? DID YOU KNOW?

Researchers at Brown University[14] found that women who exercised vigorously while trying to quit smoking were twice as likely to quit smoking and gained half as much weight as their peers who did not participate in the exercise program. Researchers are now studying the effects of moderate-intensity physical activity as an aide for smoking cessation.

Fight or Flight

All of us have experienced the symptoms of acute stress in response to a feeling of danger, whether we're startled by a loud and unexpected noise or suddenly feel threatened by someone approaching on the street. Our hearts start pounding, our blood pressure jumps, our perception narrows to a sharp focus, and we may even break into a sweat. Confronted with danger, our bodies are preparing for fight or flight. The fight or flight reaction no doubt saved our Paleolithic ancestors' lives when a wild animal suddenly threatened. Even now the response may be a lifesaver. If you have to get out of the way of a speeding car, after all, it's important to move quickly and deliberately.

However, for most stressful situations we face today—whether we're caught in a traffic jam or having a confrontation with a coworker—the fight or flight response isn't appropriate. We're not going to haul off and punch that coworker, nor are we going to run away. Still, the surge of adrenaline and the sharp rise in blood pressure, especially if they are repeated often, strain the body. This can use energy and lead to nervous tension, sleeplessness, lowered immunity, and susceptibility to conditions such as high blood pressure, migraine or tension headaches, and depression.

ACTIVITY ALERT

Stress Test

Are you under stress? Part of the answer depends on the pressures you feel at work and at home, but part of the answer also has to do with how you respond to those pressures. Here are eight true or false questions that will help you gauge whether you deal with stress in a healthy or potentially unhealthy way. Imagine how you would react in these hypothetical situations.

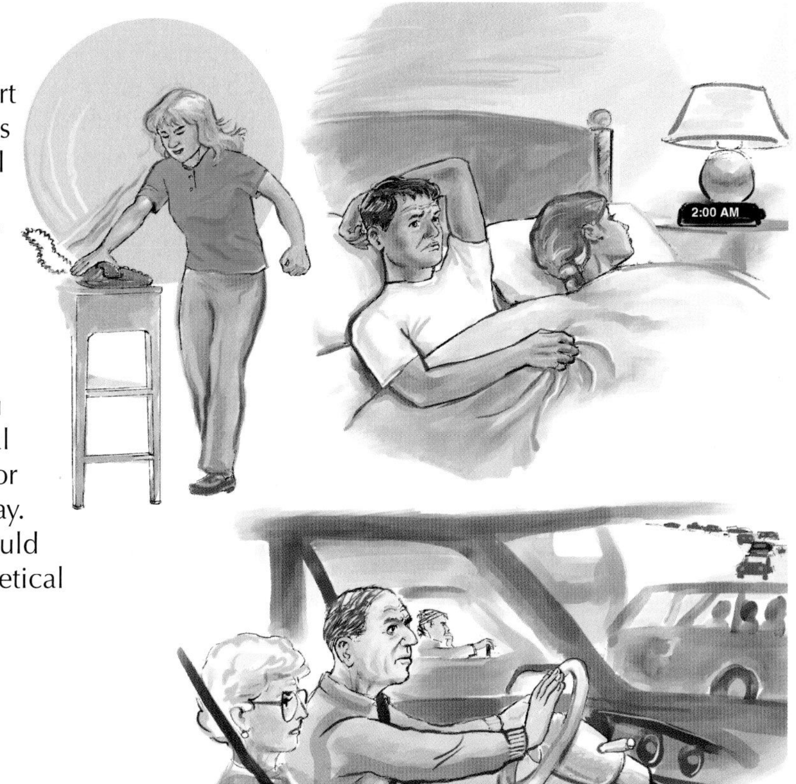

What stresses you out?

STRESS TEST

		True	False
1.	The cable repair company promised to arrive between 1:00 and 3:00, and here it is almost 4:00. You've called twice, only to get a recorded message. You can feel your anger rising and your heart beating faster.	**True**	**False**
2.	You have expensive tickets to a big game, and you're already running a little late. Your spouse is lingering over what coat to wear, though you've insisted twice that it's time to go. Suddenly you lose your patience and get angry.	**True**	**False**
3.	Things are a little shaky at work, and now you've been asked to come in for a meeting with your supervisor on Friday. You know you shouldn't let it get to you. Still, you can't help but be anxious. For the next two nights, you find yourself waking up with a feeling of dread.	**True**	**False**
4.	You've waited almost half an hour for a table at a restaurant, and suddenly the host seems to be seating a party that arrived after yours. You feel your face burn and your muscles tense up with anger.	**True**	**False**
5.	In the middle of a phone conversation, a friend gets another call on call waiting and puts you on hold. Thirty seconds pass. With your anger mounting, you slam down the phone.	**True**	**False**
6.	It's been a long, hectic day, and you know you should take some time to relax and unwind, but you can't seem to slow down. Driving home, another driver almost cuts you off by mistake. You blast the horn and hold it down long enough to show how angry you are.	**True**	**False**

In each hypothetical situation, there are different ways to respond when something goes wrong. You can get mad when a driver inadvertently cuts you off, for instance, or you can shrug it off, reminding yourself that you've done the same thing sometimes. You can slam down the phone, or you can wait until your friend gets back on the line, then gently say you'd rather have her call you back than put you on hold.

Look back over your answers. If you answered true to most questions, chances are you're what psychologists call a hot reactor. Instead of staying cool when problems arise, your heart rate accelerates, your muscles tense up, and you feel your anger surging. The more times you answered true, the more important it is to find healthy ways to defuse stress.

EXPERT ADVICE

Coping With Stress

There are many ways to let off steam. Not all of them work for everyone. The important thing is to find a strategy that works well for you. Here are some great ways to cope.

Take a Walk—or a Swim or a Bike Ride

No, we don't mean you should turn your back on stressful situations. Our point is that walking, running, bicycling, swimming, dancing, and other physical activities are some of the best stress busters around. They are a great way to unwind and blow off steam. Physical activity also has other, long-lasting benefits. Consistent moderate to vigorous physical activity, for example, can lower your heart rate. Studies of people who have lowered their heart rates have found that these individuals have lower heart rate responses during and after mental stress than people who have not been consistently active. Other studies of activity and stress show that stress hormone levels are lower during a bout of physical activity in people who are fit compared with those who are unfit. In addition to reducing the physical responses to stress, physical activity can improve mood and reduce symptoms of anxiety and depression.

Relax, the Professional Way

Another good technique is called progressive relaxation, or deep muscle relaxation. Why concentrate on muscles? Because muscles communicate with nerves and nerves directly connect to the brain. By relaxing the muscles, you can calm the mind. To practice this technique, sit in a chair or lie on a bed, and start with your hands, tensing and relaxing each muscle

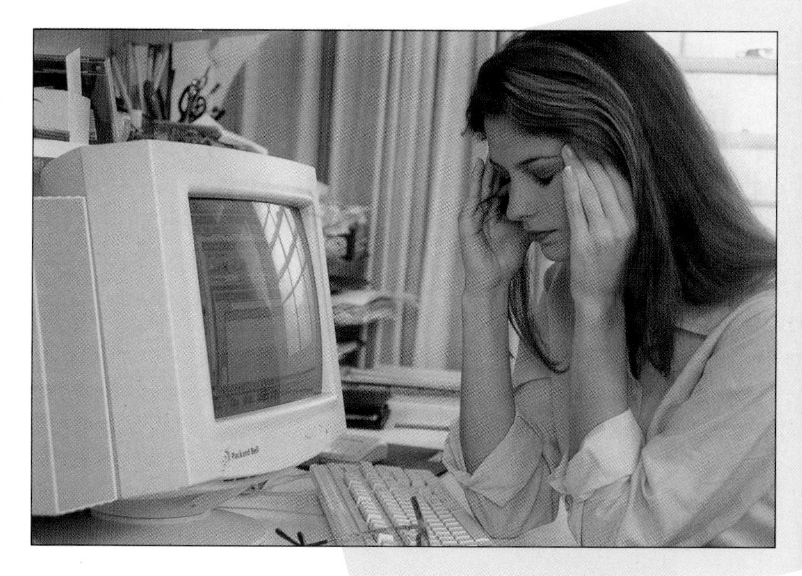

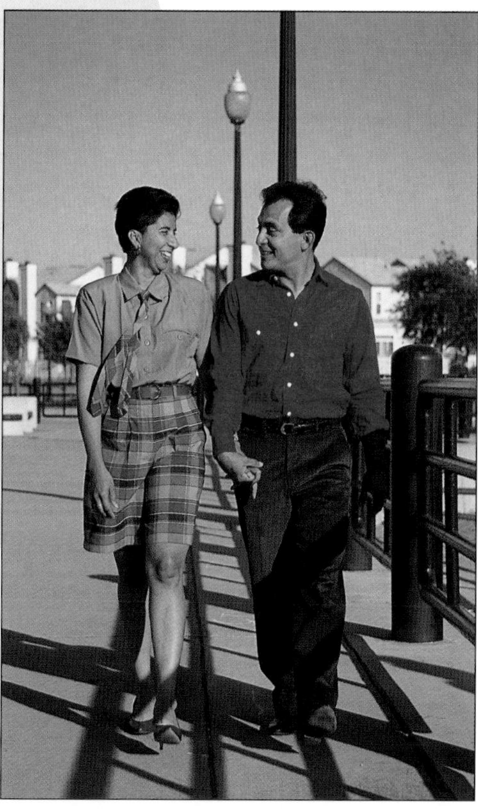

Walking and progressive relaxation can help ease stress.

group at least twice while inhaling and exhaling deeply and slowly. Next move to the muscles of your shoulders. Tense, relax, tense, and relax while inhaling and exhaling. Try the muscles in your face, or wherever you can feel the tension build. As you become skilled at this, you'll be able to tense and relax your muscles and reduce stress quickly when it occurs. You can use this stress buster even when you're sitting at your desk or behind the wheel in a traffic jam.

Use Your Imagination

A technique called imagery can also help ease the mind. It's simple: just imagine yourself in a setting where you are perfectly relaxed. It could be a mountain meadow with a stream bubbling by, or perhaps your favorite spot on earth is a beach with the surf whispering nearby, or a garden with birds singing and the smell of roses. You choose. What's important is thinking of a restful, relaxing, supportive place. Try to involve all five senses—the feel of the sun on your face, the smells carried on the breeze, the sounds of nature, the color of the leaves and flowers, or the taste of crisp, cool mountain stream water. As you feel your body beginning to relax, breathe deeply, inhaling and exhaling. Stay in your imaginary spot for 5 or 10 minutes and you'll feel the tension of the day fade away.

Have a Laugh

Anything that makes you laugh also reduces stress. A good laugh relaxes muscles and stimulates the production of stress-relieving chemicals in the brain. Watch a favorite movie comedy or television show that is usually good for a laugh, or schedule time to get together for conversation with friends you find entertaining.

? DID YOU KNOW?

Laughter may be good medicine. In a study conducted at Loma Linda University,[15] researchers divided volunteers into two groups. One group viewed a 60-minute humor video and the other group did not. Blood tests to measure biochemical changes in hormones involved in a person's response to stress, showed that the video watchers had improved levels of the hormones. This suggests that laughter may help reduce the harmful ways in which our body naturally responds to stress.

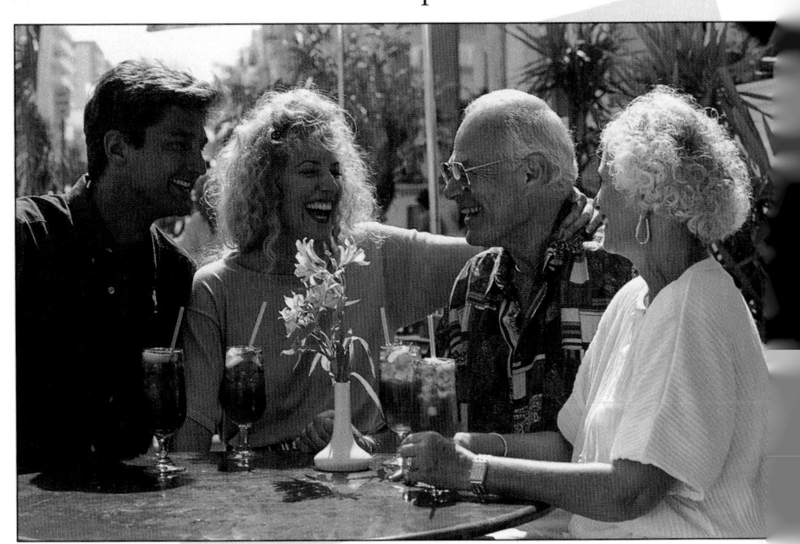

Laughter is good medicine!

UP CLOSE & PERSONAL

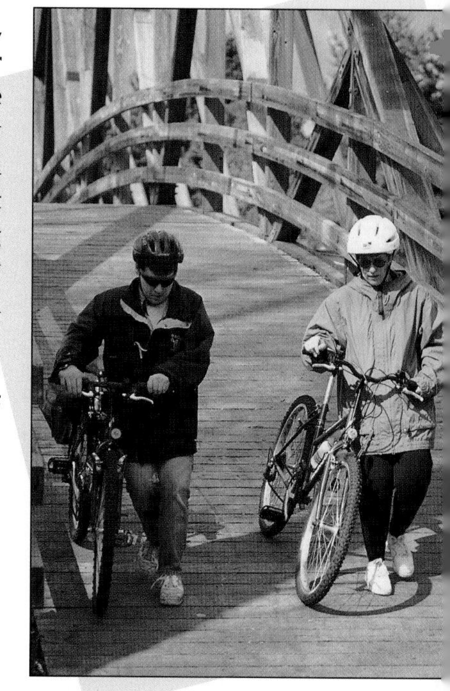

If type A people are high-pressure, hard-driven types, Rosa figured she must be type AAA. The owner of her own company, she worked long hours and had little patience for anything that got in her way. She knew she was quick to lose her temper and could be hard on her employees. She didn't realize how stressed out she'd become until she had a car accident driving home from the office one night. Annoyed at the heavy traffic and angry because she was late, she'd been following the car ahead too closely, driving too fast. When the traffic ahead came to a sudden stop, she couldn't brake in time and rear-ended the car ahead of her.

That was it, she told herself. It was time to cool off. Rosa bought a book about stress reduction techniques and tried a few. Given her nature, meditation and imagery just made her feel as if she was wasting time. When she read that physical activity can relieve stress, she decided to give it a try. She could stand to lose a few pounds, and her doctor had been hounding her about getting exercise. For half an hour at noon, she either walked or took her bike out for a spin on a nearby bike path. Gradually she began to notice that she wasn't getting as steamed up as she used to. The muscles in her back and shoulders no longer felt so tense. She also noticed that she was beginning to look forward to getting a little exercise over the noon hour just for the pleasure of it. She knew things were changing for the better when her employees got together and gave her a joke present for her birthday: handlebar streamers for her bike. ▌

EXPERT ADVICE

Stress-Busting Tips

We've already looked at some useful techniques to ease stress. Here are a few other ways to handle the pressures of daily life without turning yourself inside out:

Deal with the cause. It often helps to know what's causing you stress. You may not be able to change it completely, but you can find ways to relax things a little. If a bad relationship with your boss is stressing you out, consider one or two changes you could make to ease the situation without killing your boss. Sometimes all it takes is thinking about the situation differently.

Call on your support troops. Talking with someone helps ease any kind of stress or strain. You may even get some good advice on how to deal with the problems or pressure you're experiencing.

Take care of yourself. When you're feeling run down, things often look worse than they are, and your ability to cope may be hindered. It's important at a time like that to get enough sleep, eat a healthy diet with at least five

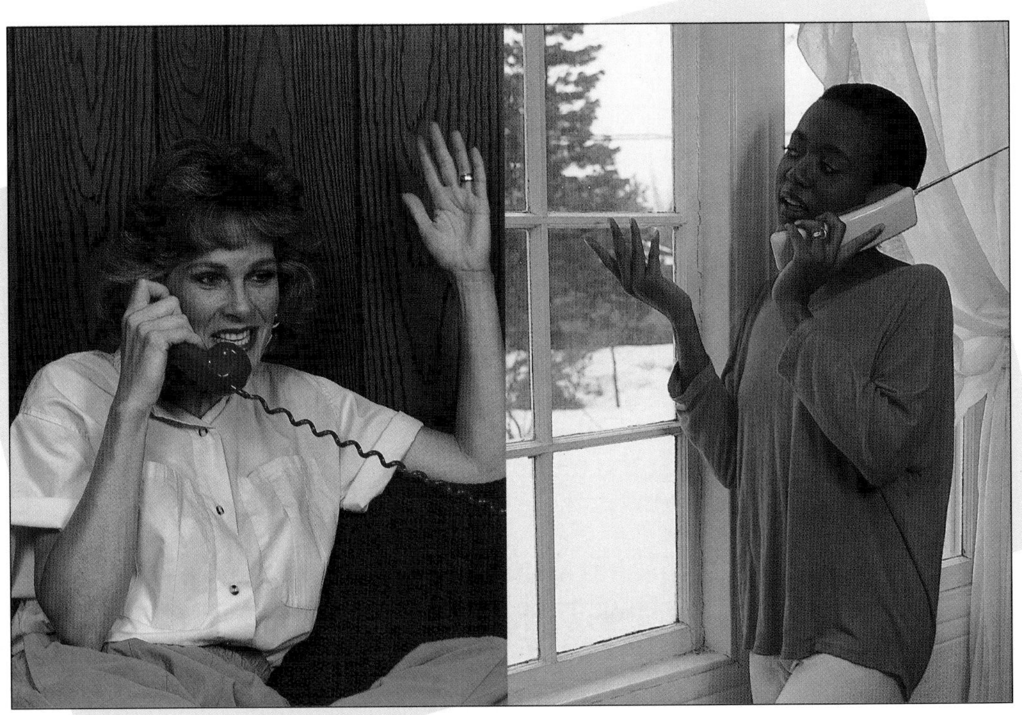

Talking with someone about your stress can help to ease it.

servings of fruits and vegetables a day, and do something nice for yourself regularly.

Take one thing at a time. Sometimes our lives are so crowded and hectic that we feel overwhelmed by the sheer number of demands on us. That's when it's important to stop, take a deep breath, and set realistic short-term goals. Put things that are most important to you at the top of the list. Take pride in what you accomplish. Be sure to give yourself a pat on the back now and then.

Learn to worry constructively. It never pays to worry for the sake of worrying. Instead, think about constructive ways to deal with the stresses in your life. One approach that often helps is to think about the problem as if it were someone else's, not your own—say your Uncle Fred's or your Aunt Minnie's. How would you advise them? Then consider taking your own advice.

Accept things you cannot change. There's nothing worse than banging your head against a wall that just won't move. Unfortunately, there are plenty of things in life we can't change, but we can change the way we think about them.

ACTIVITY ALERT

My Plan for Reducing Stress

We've looked at a variety of ways to reduce stress. Now it's time to give them a try. This week, along with your plans for everyday activities, experiment with at least two stress-busting techniques. Just to show you we mean business, we're going to ask you to put your plan in writing. Write down two ways of coping with stress that you'll try this week. For example, you might get some additional physical activity and try progressive muscle relaxation or you might rent a funny movie or try imagery. Be aware of how you're feeling before, during, and after each technique.

Two stress-reducing techniques to try this week

1.____

2.____

How well did 1 work? (Circle one.)

Very well Moderately well Not at all

How well did 2 work? (Circle one.)

Very well Moderately well Not at all

If these two techniques didn't help you let off steam, try another. If the strategies you tried worked moderately well, give yourself more time to practice them. Even relaxing doesn't always come easy. Some people have to practice a while before they get the hang of it.

If you answered "very well," congratulations. Now write down some situations when you plan to use them (when work is hectic, for instance, or after a long day, when the kids are in bed and the house is finally quiet).

____

____

ACTIVITY ALERT

What Progress Have You Made?

You've reached the end of week 13. To monitor your progress toward making a lasting change, take another moment to check your readiness to change. Be honest. Once you're done, look back at your previous responses (weeks 2, 5, and 9) to see how you've changed over the past three months. Remember, appendix B provides helpful tips for each stage of readiness.

By now, we hope, you can see yourself making progress. Even if you haven't come quite as far as you'd like, you've made a big step by getting this far. As we've said before, some people need to remain at one stage longer than others before they move on. In our studies at Brown University, we have learned that taking longer to move through the stages doesn't mean you will end up less successful than someone who moves through them more quickly. By going at your own pace, you'll have a good chance of making a lasting change.

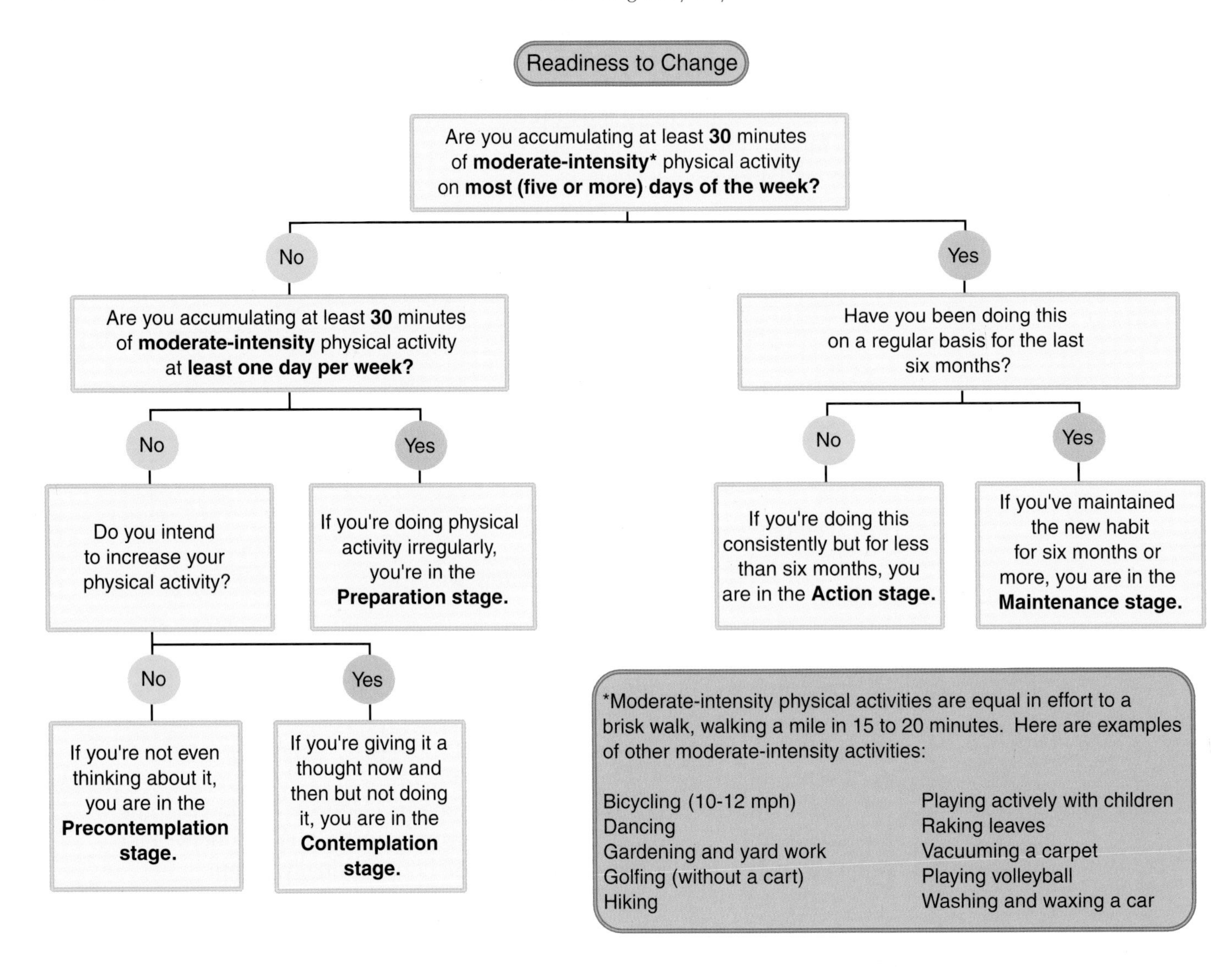

Chapter Checklist

Before you move on to the next week's activities, make sure you

- Completed your stress test to see if you are a hot reactor
- Identified ways to relax
- Made a plan for dealing with stress
- Completed the Readiness to Change form

By now you've come to understand that stress can take a serious toll on your plans for making healthful changes. You've also identified several ways to relax and defuse tension. Next week, we'll look at a high-tech way to gauge how much activity you do every step of the way.

WEEK **FOURTEEN**

Step by Step

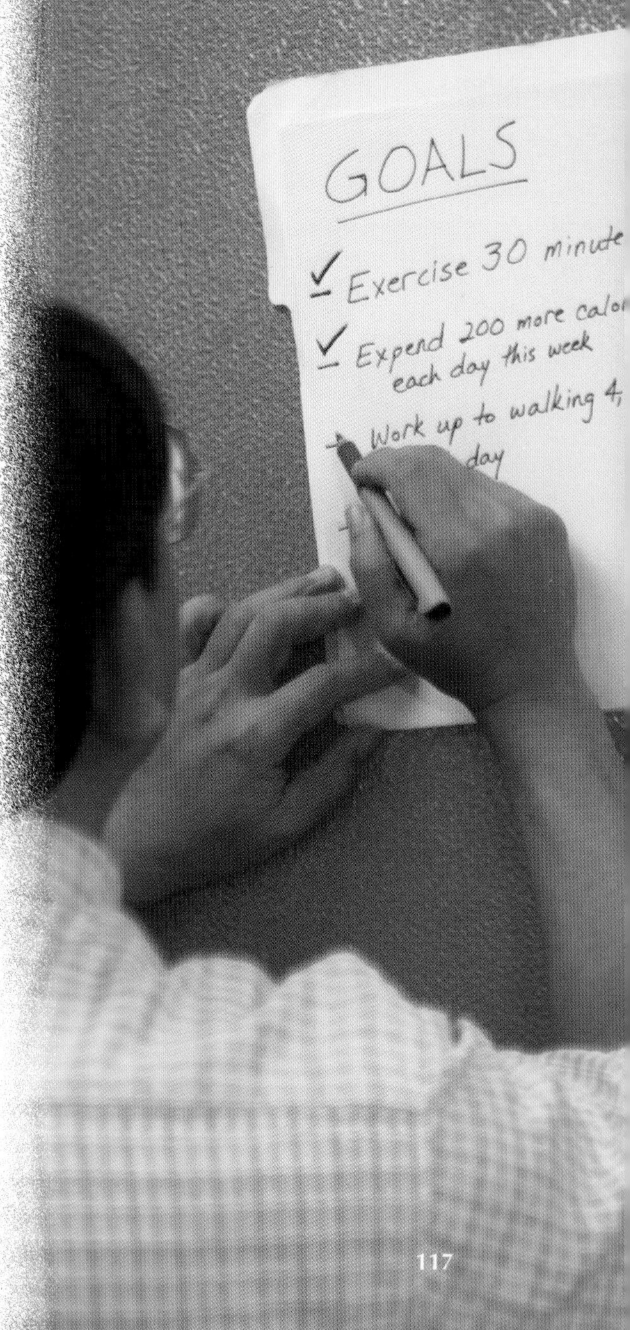

In This Chapter

- Reviewing ways to monitor activity
- Introducing the step counter
- Keeping a weekly activity log
- Setting specific goals

By now you've found plenty of opportunities to do some physical activities every day. The best part about everyday physical activity is that it becomes part of your life. Climbing the stairs instead of an escalator becomes second nature. Walking to town rather than driving becomes part of your routine. Instead of having to go to the gym, lifestyle exercisers build in activities throughout the day, often for a few minutes here, a few minutes there.

With everyday activity being accumulated in small chunks, it's tricky to monitor your progress. So this week we'll look at a few familiar ways of monitoring your activity level. We'll also introduce a new way that many participants in our programs liked best of all.

Why Monitor?

We don't need to tell you that making a lasting change in your life isn't easy. Some weeks you meet your goals; others you might fall short. It's easy to get discouraged if you're looking at only the small picture.

That's why monitoring your progress is so important. By monitoring your activity level week by week, you can keep track of the large picture. You can also look back over a rocky period and understand the obstacles that got in your way.

EXPERT ADVICE

Ways to Track Your Activity

By now you've tried a variety of ways to monitor your activity. One approach is to add up the time you spend doing physical activities that are at least moderately strenuous. That method works well if your goal is to do at least 30 minutes of activity every day.

Another way to monitor activity is to calculate the number of calories you expend. That approach is gratifying if your goal is not only to add activity but also to lose weight.

In our studies at The Cooper Institute and at Brown University, we introduced participants to another way of measuring activity—devices called step counters. We were surprised at how popular they proved to be. Step counters are little devices that you can attach to a belt. Equipped with a mechanical pendulum, they record every step you take. They're a great way to keep track of how much activity you do every day. They can also help you set goals for doing even more.

Selecting a Step Counter

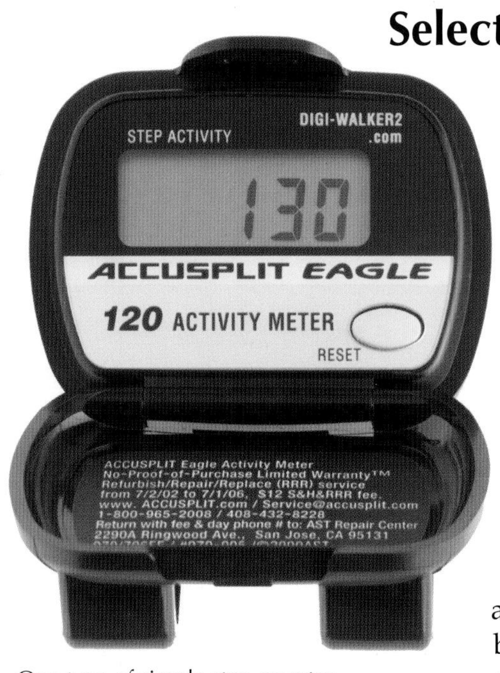

One type of simple step counter.

If you took our advice in week 6, you should already have your step counter. If not, you can easily find a good one at your local sports store. There are several versions. Some simply count steps. Others come equipped with all sorts of bells and whistles.

We recommend buying one that simply counts steps. Devices that promise to convert steps into distances like miles usually aren't accurate. That's because you have to program in how long your stride is. But throughout the day not every step you take is precisely the same length. Step counters that convert activity into calories expended aren't accurate either, because they can't distinguish between activities that are different in intensity.

Simple step counters, on the other hand, are reliable, as several good studies have shown. The model we prefer and the one we use in our programs is the Digi-Walker brand. Here's how you can order the Digi-Walker step counter:

New Lifestyles
5900 Larson Avenue
Kansas City, MO 64133
888-748-5377
www.digiwalker.com

Accusplit
2290A Ringwood Avenue
San Jose, CA 95131-1718
800-935-1996
www.accusplit.com

How to Use Your Step Counter

Step counters contain a small pendulum that moves each time you step. For the greatest accuracy, keep your step counter centered over your right or left hipbone. This should line up where the front crease of your trousers would be.

The step counter *must* be firmly attached. The best bet is to wear it on a belt. Another option is to attach it to the waistband of gym shorts, pantyhose, or underwear.

A note for those who wear the step counter on your underwear or pantyhose: Put the step counter inside the band not outside the band of your garment. Be sure to remove it before you use the toilet. Otherwise you might need to go fishing. We have discovered even if they get wet, once they dry out, they still work!

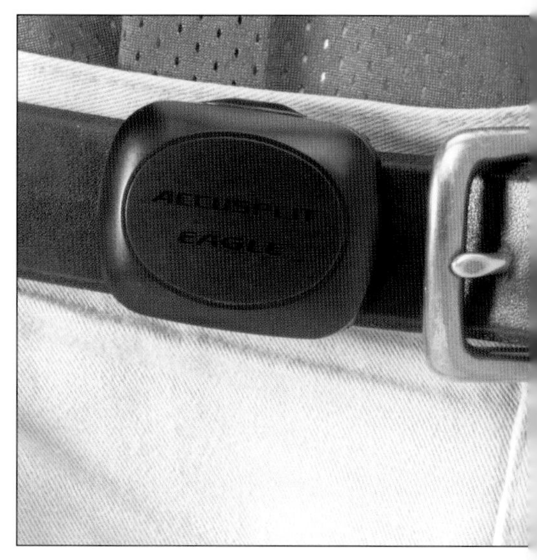

Attach the step counter to your belt or waistband, centered over your right or left hipbone.

ACTIVITY ALERT

Establish Your Starting Line

First, use the step counter to calculate how many steps you typically take during the day. Attach the step counter to your belt as soon as you get dressed, and keep it on until you're ready to go to bed. At the end of the day or before you get started the next morning, record how many steps you took. Be sure to reset your step counter at the beginning of each new day.

Wear it every day for a week and keep track of your steps. Use the forms on the next page. An extra blank copy is included in appendix D. Make a few photocopies of that page so you'll have plenty of activity logs. From our experience, most inactive people tally between 2,000 and 4,000 steps just going about their everyday business.

STEP-BY-STEP

WEEKLY ACTIVITY LOG

Week: ______________________

Day of week	Date	Step goal	Actual steps	Minutes of activity Moderate	Hard	Notes
Monday						
Tuesday						
Wednesday						
Thursday						
Friday						
Saturday						
Sunday						

Week: ______________________

Day of week	Date	Step goal	Actual steps	Minutes of activity Moderate	Hard	Notes
Monday						
Tuesday						
Wednesday						
Thursday						
Friday						
Saturday						
Sunday						

EXPERT ADVICE

Setting Specific Goals

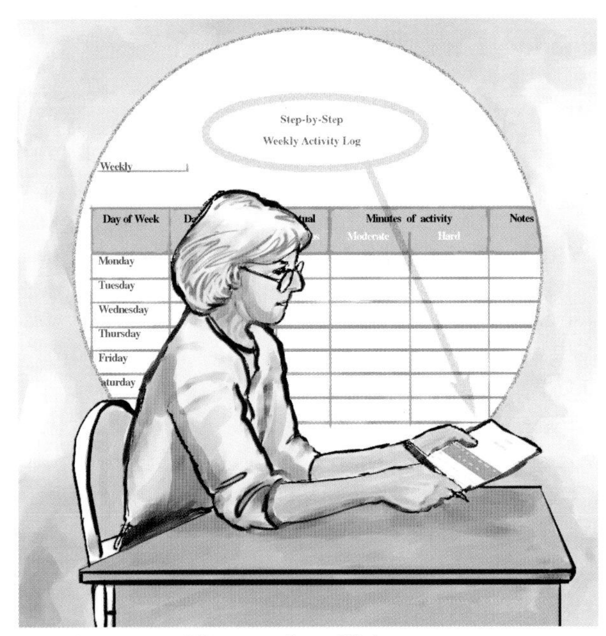

Setting specific goals will improve your chances of success.

Studies of behavior change all come to the same commonsense conclusion: the more specific your goal, the more likely you are to reach it. It's not enough to say, "I'm going to try to eat a healthier diet." To make that happen, you've got to get specific.

That's where step counters come in handy. They're a great way not only to monitor your progress but also to set goals for yourself. Our studies at The Cooper Institute have found that participants who set specific goals, then kept track of their activity were the most successful at improving their overall fitness, losing weight, and decreasing their blood pressure.

Step It Up

Daily Step Goal

Shoot for getting 10,000 or more steps per day.

After you have recorded your steps for a week, calculate your average steps per day. Next, set a reasonable goal to increase the average number of steps you take. If you typically take 4,000 steps, set a goal of 4,500 a day. Once you get there, raise the bar again. The ultimate goal should be about 10,000 steps each day. Our research shows that if you accumulate this many steps every day, chances are good you're getting many basic benefits of physical activity. If you are trying to lose weight you will need to do more, say 12,000 to 15,000 steps a day.

DID YOU KNOW?

- Walking for 30 minutes at a brisk pace equals approximately 2,500 to 3,500 steps. How many steps do *you* get by walking briskly for half an hour?
- Walking briskly during the four minutes of commercials between shows can tally up approximately 350 to 400 steps. How many steps can you take during commercials for your favorite TV program?

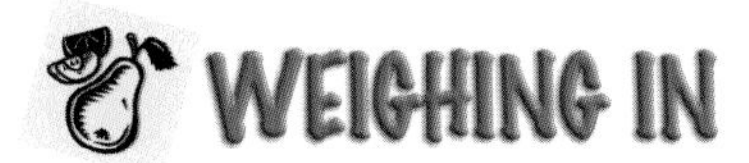

Losing Weight Takes Time

- The more active you are, the more muscle mass you will have.
- By increasing muscle mass, you increase your strength and fitness.
- Physical activity leads to reducing body fat, lowering blood pressure, and lowering cholesterol levels.
- Getting fit is as important as weight loss and may be more so.
- Make physical activity, not losing weight, your first priority.

Don't Be Pound Foolish

One leading reason most people resolve to become active is to lose weight. No wonder. Recent studies suggest that more than half of Americans are overweight.

However, a goal of losing a set number of pounds can mean trouble. For starters, it's easy to get discouraged. Losing weight takes time. When the pounds don't fall off over a few weeks, many people give up. It's important to remember, too, that when you become active, you increase the amount of muscle mass in your body. So even if your weight on the scale remains the same, healthy changes are taking place. You're replacing fat with muscle. and muscle weighs more than fat.

Our studies have shown that increasing physical activity, even when people don't lose weight, results in important health benefits, such as losing body fat and lowering both blood pressure and cholesterol levels. We recently studied whether being physically fit protected overweight men from dying prematurely.[16] We found that men who were obese but fit had a much lower risk of dying prematurely than obese men who were unfit. Astonishingly, we found that obese, fit men had a lower risk of dying prematurely than even the lean but unfit men! Preliminary data from The Cooper Institute suggest the same association is true for women. If you want to lose weight, fine. Just make sure that's not your only goal. Remember that there are plenty of other excellent benefits you get from becoming physically active.

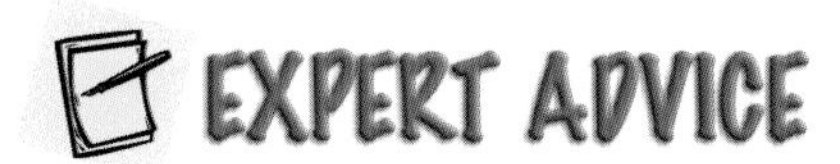

Electronic Coach

Wouldn't it be great to have a personal coach? Someone who was there to tell you how you're doing and encourage you when you slump?

Step counters can be the next best thing. From time to time during the day, check to see how many steps you've taken. If it's already midafternoon and you've tallied only 1,500 steps, it's time to get moving. Take an activity coffee break, or get off the bus a few stops early and walk the rest of the way home. Use your step counter to monitor your progress during the day and to encourage you to push a little harder than yesterday. The one-day record for a participant in Project *Active* was 36,000 steps!

UP CLOSE & PERSONAL

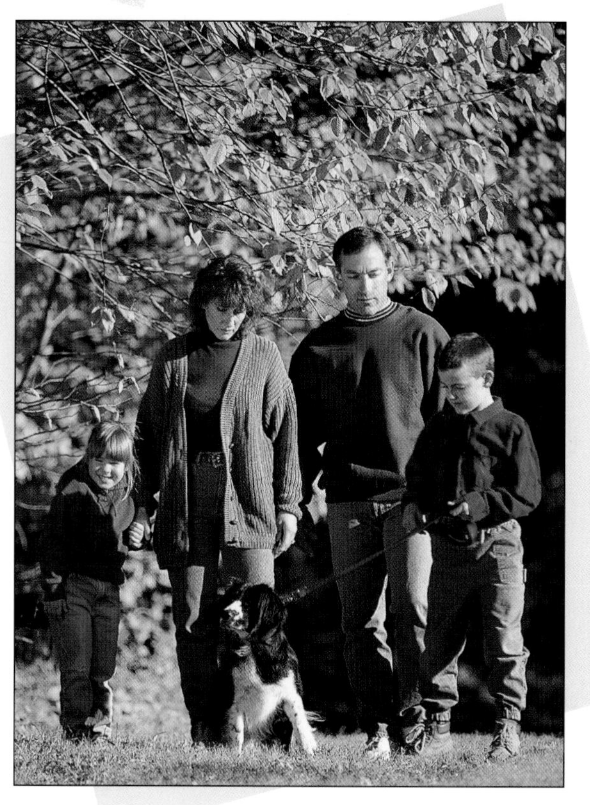

As much as she tried, Jeannine never seemed to be able to stick with the program. Adding up the minutes spent climbing stairs or walking in from the far end of the parking lot seemed too complicated. Given her schedule at the office and home, setting aside the same time for a 15-minute walk every day just didn't work either. Never knowing whether she'd met her goal, she began to feel discouraged.

That was before she tried the step counter. The first day out, she was gratified to discover the few changes she'd already made added up to 6,000 steps a day. Encouraged, she decided to add 1,000 steps. Before work, she and her husband would set out to walk until she'd reached 1,000. Then she would add another 6,000 steps through her daily activities. The time spent walking was so pleasant that it wasn't long before Jeannine was averaging 10,000 steps a day. She got her husband a step counter too, and they had fun competing to see who could tally up the most steps.

Soon the whole family got into the act. Their teenage sons wanted step counters, and they all began to post their totals on a magnetic calendar on the refrigerator. Whoever won got to pick a place for a dinner out on the weekend.

NEED A BOOST?

Are you having a hard time keeping up? You're not alone. Making a lasting change in your life, whether it's becoming active or adopting a healthy diet, takes time. Sometimes you'll take a step backward. That's the time to remind yourself that the benefits are worth the effort and resolve to take two steps forward. Here are some tips that may help:

- Modify your expectations and goals to make sure they are reasonable. Remember, Rome wasn't built in a day.
- Plan ahead for situations that may sabotage your efforts. Think of ways to deal with these obstacles before they knock you off track.
- Getting bored or stale are two common reasons people lose interest in physical activity. If that's the way you feel, push yourself to try one or two new activities, or find a new setting for the activities you love.
- Choose how to reward yourself in a special way for meeting your next important goal.
- Don't feel guilty if you haven't met your goals. Guilt only makes the problem seem worse than it is. Instead of moping, go for a brisk 10-minute walk. Then plan ways to add at least 30 minutes of activity each day for the next three days.

This week, you've used a step counter to calculate how many steps you typically take each day. You may find that a step counter does more than just keep track of your activities. If you're like many participants in our programs, you'll also find that these nifty devices encourage you to push yourself a little harder than yesterday.

Chapter Checklist

Before you move on to the next week's activities, make sure you

- Learned to use your step counter
- Filled in the Step-by-Step Weekly Activity Log
- Set a goal for increasing the number of steps you take each day

Sneaking in more time for activities isn't always easy. Remember the advertisements for automatic appliances that were predicted to make our lives easier and give us more time than doing things the old way? In many ways they have made our lives easier, but somehow most of us feel more rushed than ever. All of us wonder how we'll find the time to do everything we need and want to do. During the next week we'll look at effective ways to manage our time.

WEEK **FIFTEEN**

Managing Your Time

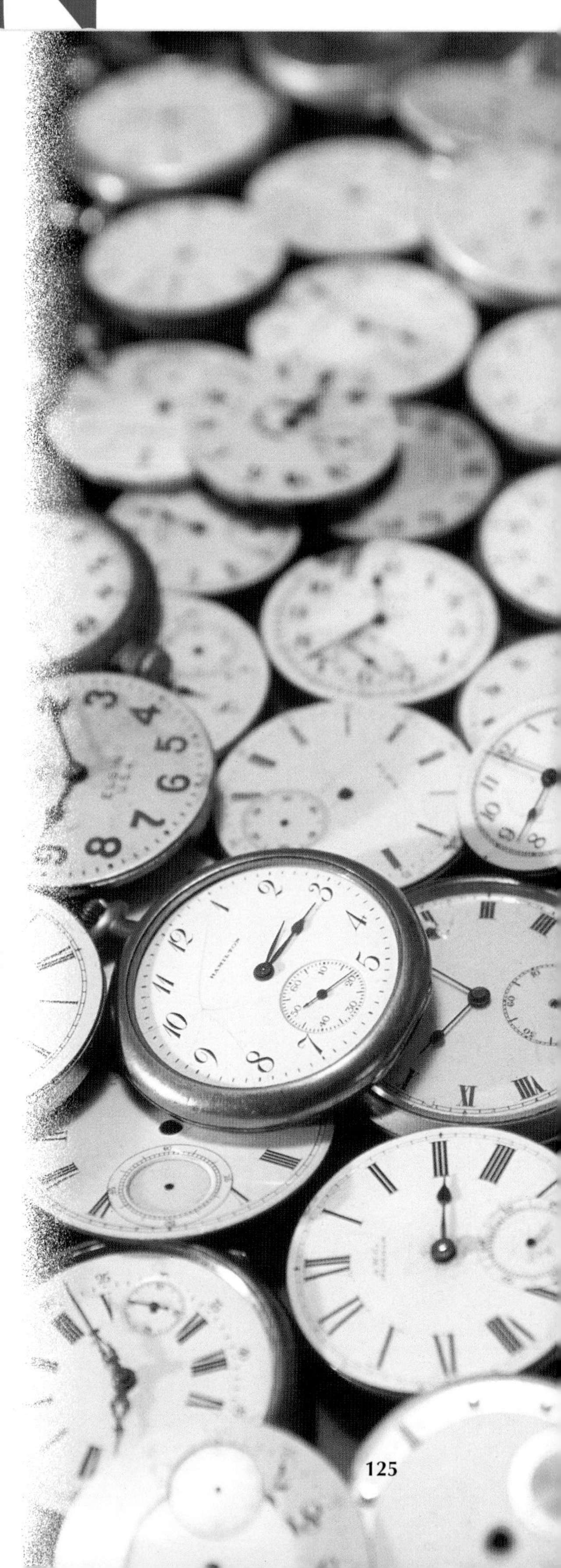

In This Chapter

- Setting priorities
- Finding the time in your busy schedule
- Identifying time squeezers

If you're like most people, you probably wish there were 25 hours in the day, so you'd have time to do all the things you need and want to do. Not having enough time, in fact, is the biggest reason most people say they don't get enough physical activity.

Well, we're stuck with 24 hours in the day, whether we like it or not. It's up to us to decide how to use that time. We can't do away with some demands in our lives, such as work and family responsibilities, but we *can* manage them more wisely than we do. All of us, no matter how hectic our schedules are, have time we can spend any way we choose. This week we'll look at how to make sure you have time to do what matters.

Setting Priorities

With so many demands competing for time, the first thing we need to do is set priorities. What are the things we value? What are the things we most want to accomplish? One handy way is to make a list of the things you do each day. Then rate the different activities using a four-point scale, with 1 being the things you value highly and 4 being things you don't value. Here's what a sample priority list of activities might look like:

1	2	3	4
Value highly	Value somewhat	Neutral	Don't value

Task	Value
Read the newspaper	3
Taught classes	1
Wrote report	2
Walked at lunch	1
Met with parents	1
Played with children	1
Cleaned house	2
Watched television	4
Talked to friends on telephone	3

A quick glance over those priorities makes it clear which activities matter and which don't. Anything that ranks a 4—watching television in this example—you can easily replace with something that matters more (such as getting out and walking for half an hour). You don't necessarily have to replace one task with another. You can borrow a little time from one to devote to another. In this case, you could decide to give up some of the time now spent reading the paper to take a 15-minute walk after breakfast. Another option is to combine tasks—to turn time with friends into activity by suggesting walking together rather than talking on the telephone.

ACTIVITY ALERT

My Priorities

Now take a few minutes to think about the tasks you did yesterday. Include everything that required 15 minutes or more of your time. Then give each activity a value from 1 to 4. Be honest with yourself about the priority each activity has in your mind. The only activities that score a 1 should be ones that *really* matter to you.

WHAT MATTERS?

1	2	3	4
Value highly	Value somewhat	Neutral	Don't value

Task	Value

Taking time to exercise does not mean giving up what is important to you.

Look back at your list. If your list is predominantly 1s and 2s, you're doing the things that matter most to you and are managing your time well. If your list includes more 3s and 4s, chances are you may feel frustrated and stressed because you're not doing what matters most. No one wants to fill his or her day with activities they don't care about. If that sounds like you, it's time to use a few problem-solving strategies to figure out how to spend more time doing the things you value most.

EXPERT ADVICE

Who's in Charge Here Anyway?

In week 13 we looked at few ways to fight stress. Here's another useful tip. Compared with people who feel frazzled when things get stressful, stress-hardy people seem to have three important attitudes—the three Cs of surviving stress: challenge, commitment, and control. Stress-hardy individuals

- see change as a *challenge*, not a threat;
- feel a strong *commitment* to their jobs, their families, and their decision to change; and
- have a firm sense of *control* over their lives and how they spend their time.

The third C is one reason time management is so important. By gaining control over how you spend the time you have, you'll lower stress and increase self-confidence. You'll also feel at the end of the day that you've accomplished what *really* matters to you.

UP CLOSE & PERSONAL

Marcus began each week full of good intentions, but by midweek he was skipping his walk over the noon hour because something else always came up. When he sat down to list all the things he needed and wanted to do, he realized how crowded his day was, with work, the kids, the house, and all the other demands. Most of the time he didn't feel as if he had much control over his schedule.

My Priorities
1 Help kids with homework
2 Work hard for promotion
3 Family bike ride this weekend
4 Volunteer at favorite charity
5 Be active for 30 minutes, 5 days per week
PUT GARBAGE OUT!
Phone Directory

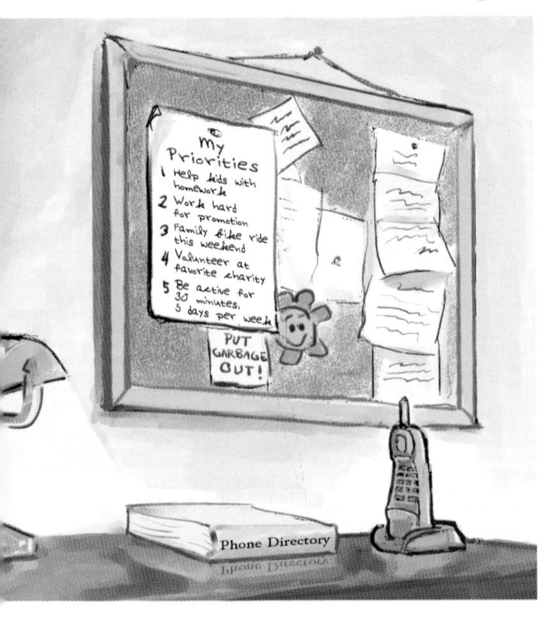

Looking at how he spent his time was a revelation for Marcus. He realized that not all the demands on his time were equally important, nor did he place the same value on them. Once the kids were in bed, Marcus and his wife had gotten into the habit of stretching out on the sofa and watching television. But there were only two programs Marcus enjoyed. Sometimes it was impossible to get away over the lunch hour. If he made walking for half an hour a top priority, however, he realized he could usually do that *and* get his work done.

So Marcus changed his activity plan to make better use of his time. He set a goal of walking at least three days a week during the noon hour. That allowed for two days off if his schedule became too hectic. He and his wife agreed that on the other two nights of the week, instead of vegging on the sofa, they'd walk through the neighborhood together.

To his surprise, Marcus found that he had plenty of time to be active. The trick was making activity a top priority.

Beware the Time Squeezers

We don't need to tell you that all kinds of things can suddenly turn your best-laid plans upside down. Just when you think you have the time you need for physical activity, a time squeezer like one of the following situations comes along. Sound familiar?

- The boss piles on work.
- Someone in the family gets sick and needs attention.
- You have to run to the store for an ingredient you forgot to buy for dinner.
- Traffic is terrible and you spend an extra half hour on the highway.
- An old friend calls and wants to chat for an hour.
- The bathtub springs a leak and you need to find a plumber right away.

These things happen to all of us. That's why the concept of fitting activity in and using the step counter is *so* important. On days when you get squeezed for time, be as active as possible by taking as many steps as you can. You'll be surprised by how active you can be, even on the most hectic day.

WEIGHING IN

American Dietetic Association
800-877-1600
www.eatright.org

National Heart, Lung, and Blood Institute
www.nhlbi.nih.gov

U.S. Department of Agriculture
Center for Nutrition Policy and Promotion
www.usda.gov/cnpp

Like most health experts, we're convinced that regular physical activity is a crucial component of any weight-loss plan. Just as important, of course, is controlling the number of calories you consume. In virtually all studies, people who combine activity with a sensible eating plan are more likely to maintain weight loss than those who simply diet. The typical weight loss is in the range of 5 to 10 pounds (2.26-4.5 kg). That may not sound like a lot, but it's enough to lower the risk of heart disease and diabetes, as well as certain forms of cancer.

Not everyone who increases their activity will lose weight. People who are lean to start with don't have much fat to lose. The people most likely to lose weight are those who have been inactive and are slightly overweight.

Studies show that when people use dieting alone for weight loss, they regain most of the weight within a year or two. The best success in losing weight and keeping it off occurs in people who combine exercise with a sensible eating plan. On the left are a few good resources for learning about healthful eating.

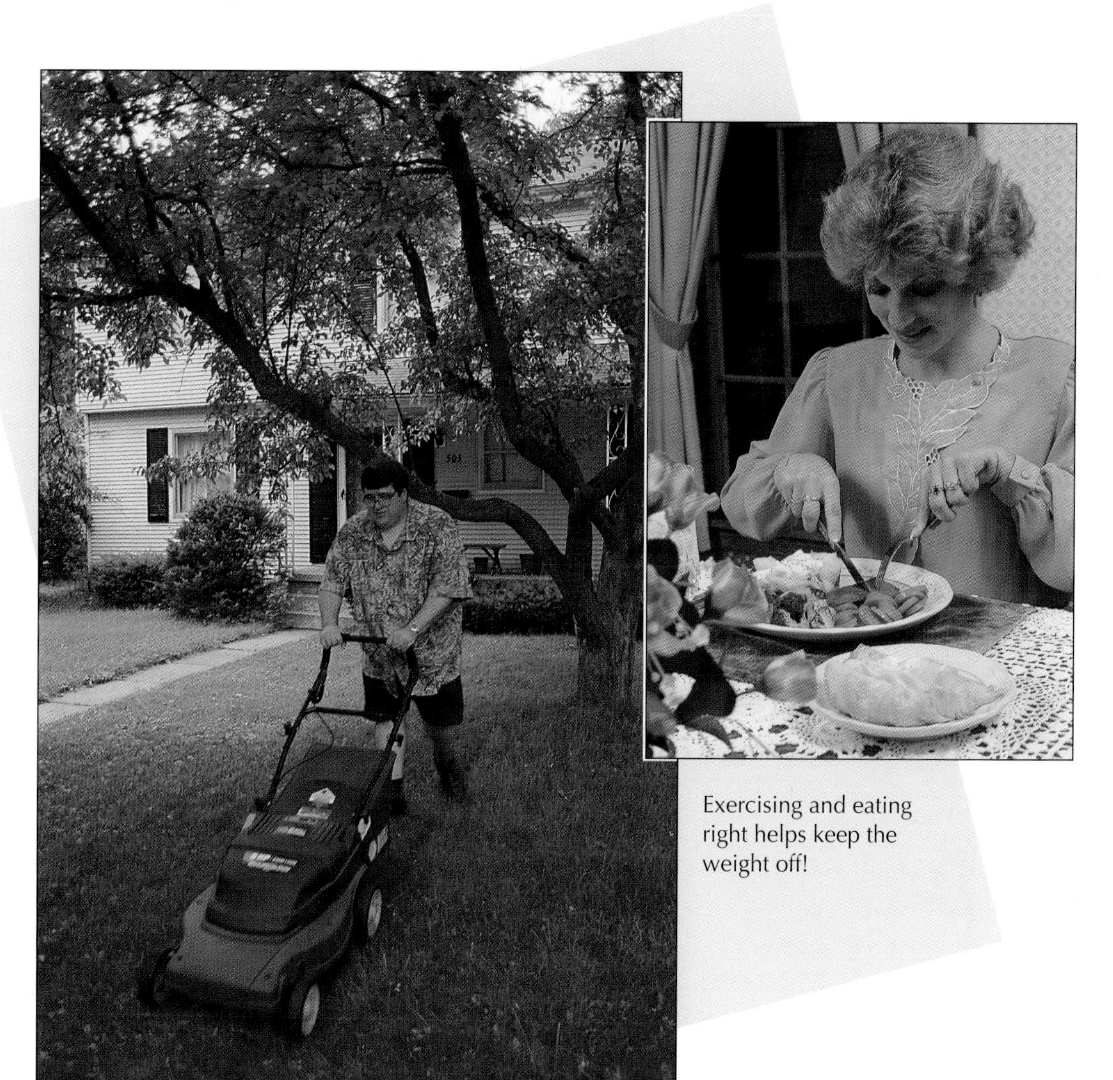

Exercising and eating right helps keep the weight off!

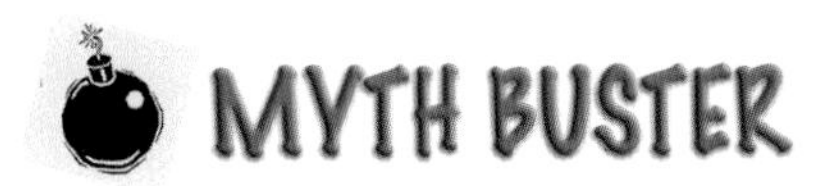

"Specific exercises can burn fat from specific areas of the body."

Magazine articles may promise to give us the secret to trimmer thighs or a flatter stomach, but those promises are misleading. Specific exercises *can* strengthen specific muscles or increase flexibility around a joint used in certain activities, but when it comes to burning calories and reducing fat, all activities are equally good. The more intense the activity and the longer you do it, the more calories you burn. It's as simple as that. Specific exercises do not slim or spot-reduce hips, thighs, or tummies.

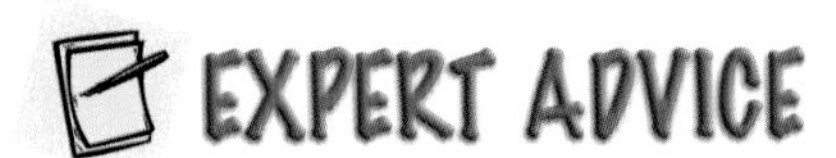

Time-Management Techniques

Managing your time goes hand in hand with setting goals. After all, if meeting a goal matters to you, you need to set aside the time to do it. That means breaking your long-term goal down into short-term goals, then thinking about what you need to do each day to achieve them. If need be, write down your physical activity goals and your current plan for achieving them. Then make sure you include them on your list of priorities for the day.

People use a variety of techniques for managing time. One effective method is to list the activities for the day that you plan to accomplish. You can do this the night before or first thing in the morning. If you prefer to plan for an entire week, write up your to-do list Sunday night or Monday morning.

Another approach is to use a calendar and assign your top-priority items a specific time during the day. That's especially important if, like most people, you are more productive or energetic at one time of day than another. For example, some people wake up in the morning ready to go and fully alert. Others may do their best work in the afternoon or evening. Put your must-do tasks in your best part of the day.

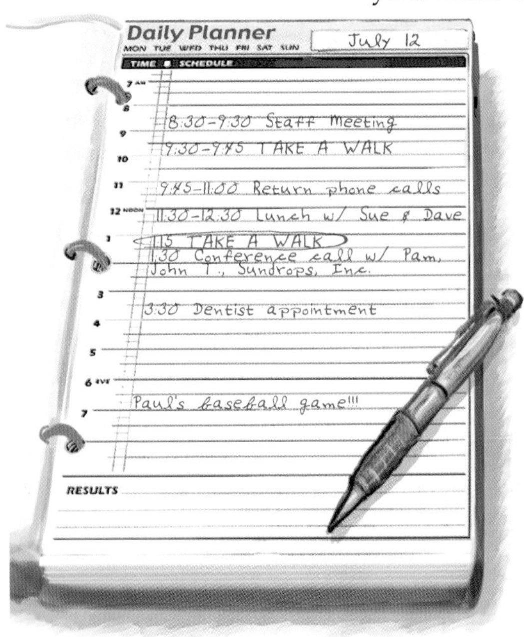

Whatever approach you choose, be realistic. After all, there's only so much any of us can accomplish in a day. Too ambitious a list will only make you frustrated and discouraged. Also, be sure to give yourself time for breaks. Physical activity can be a terrific break from desk work.

Finally, don't be discouraged if your best-laid plans get thrown off schedule. Sometimes unavoidable demands take up more time than you expected, squeezing out other tasks. At work, for instance, staff meetings often go longer than anticipated. At home, you may find that once you get started tidying up the house, you discover many things that need your attention. If you see a time squeezer on the horizon, try to schedule it for later in the day, after you've done your top-priority items (and we hope that includes physical activity).

"I Should" or "I Want To"

Take a moment to look back at your list of priorities. Chances are many top items are things you know you *should* do. One reason most people try to increase their activity is they know they should, but should only goes so far. To make any lasting change, you have to turn what you should do into something you value doing. That way you're likely to find the time to do it.

ACTIVITY ALERT

Of course, we have an ulterior motive in asking you to list your priorities. We're hoping that by now, getting at least 30 minutes of physical activity most days of the week is right up there with the *numero uno* activities of your day. We'll even settle for being number two on a day when you've got lots of other important things going on. However, if you honestly can't give activity the first or second priority in your day, you might want to look back weekly to revisit the list of benefits you hope to get from being active.

Take a moment to think about tomorrow and the coming week. What do you have to do? What do you *want* to do? Use the following space to organize your tasks into three priority categories: must do, hope to do, and do if I have time. Make the list as complete as possible. Create a list just for tomorrow if that seems appropriate, or think about the entire week.

THIS WEEK'S PRIORITIES

Date ____________________

Must do ____

____

____

Hope to do ____

____

____

Do if I have time ____

____

____

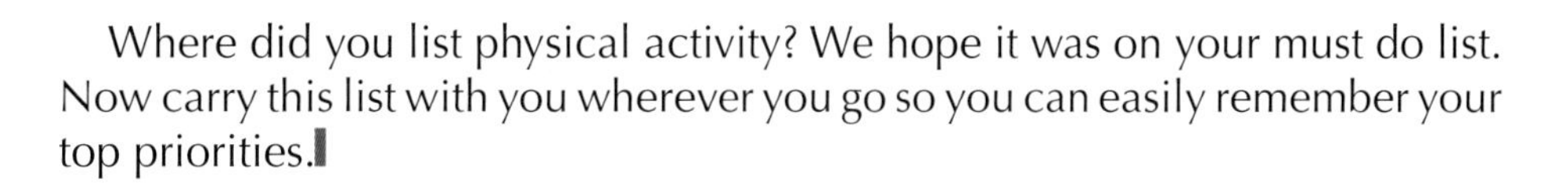

Where did you list physical activity? We hope it was on your must do list. Now carry this list with you wherever you go so you can easily remember your top priorities.

Chapter Checklist

Before you move on to the next week's activities, make sure you

- Assigned priorities to the things you need to do and want to do
- Organized the coming week's tasks according to must do, hope to do, and do if I have time
- Recognized time squeezers that often make it hard to effectively manage your time

---

By setting priorities, you'll find it easier to do the things that matter to you, including, we hope, getting physical activity. Time-management techniques are useful no matter what you want to do. If you find yourself getting frazzled because you don't have enough hours in the day, remember this week's message and use the same techniques to set priorities. Next week, we'll look at opportunities in the community for turning activity into something you look forward to doing.

WEEK SIXTEEN

Exploring New Activities

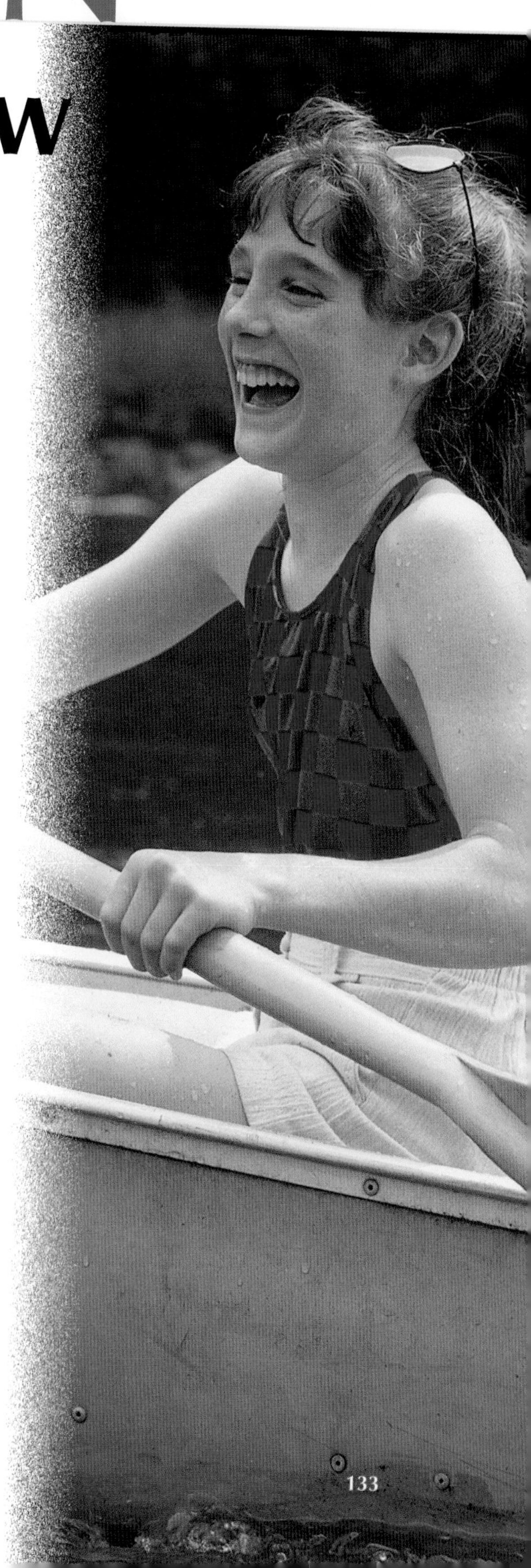

In This Chapter

- Identifying new opportunities to be physically active
- Checking out physical activity options in your community
- Selecting in-home exercise equipment

As we've said, labor-saving devices have steadily diminished opportunities for physical activity. First came cars, then washing machines and dryers, then riding mowers, each lessening the activity in our lifestyles. Now with the Home Shopping Network and the Internet we don't even need to get up from a chair to go shopping!

The result of these innovations is that we all have to work these days to be active. Luckily, there are plenty of opportunities. Over the last weeks we've already looked at a few:

Instead of	**Try**
Hiring someone to do your yard work	Doing it yourself
Driving to the store for one item	Walking or riding your bike
Going to the movies on a Saturday afternoon	Going for a bike ride or hike
Taking a lazy vacation	Enjoying an active vacation
Taking the escalator or elevator	Climbing the stairs

In this chapter we'll look at other opportunities for activity right in your backyard.

Checking Out Community Resources

Most communities have a wealth of recreational opportunities. The parks and recreation departments organize some. People who like to get together for activities such as bicycling, hiking, square dancing, or swimming form others. Most groups welcome newcomers, even people with little experience. Some examples include the following:

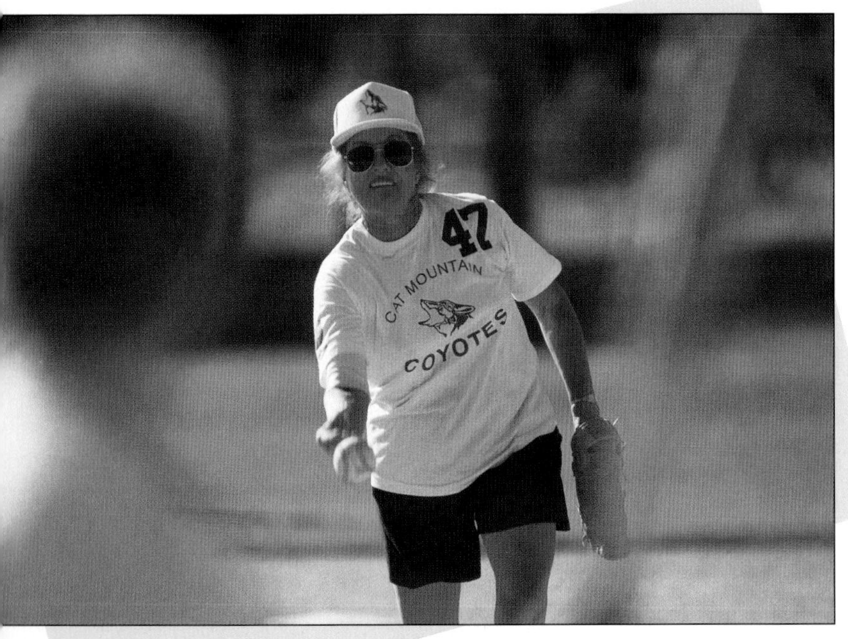

Parks and recreation departments offer a wealth of activity opportunities, even for adults.

- Cycling clubs
- Dancing clubs
- Fun runs and walks
- Golfing leagues
- In-line skating groups
- Orienteering clubs
- Outdoor clubs
- Racquetball leagues
- Rowing and canoeing clubs
- Running clubs
- Soccer leagues
- Swimming clubs
- Tennis leagues
- Volleyball leagues
- Walking clubs

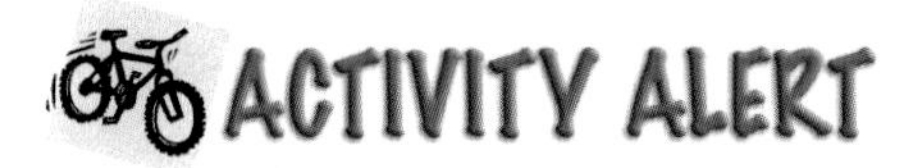

Searching for Activities

This week, check out what your community has to offer. There are many ways to get information. One place to start is your local recreation center or the parks and recreation department. The local newspaper probably lists information on recreational activities as well.

Another good source for useful information is the Internet. (If you don't have Internet access at home, chances are good you can find it at your local library.) Use one of the many search engines to find out about activities of special interest to you. You can narrow your search by adding the name of your town or county.

Of course, you can also try the old-fashioned way, by consulting a book at the local library or bookstore. Sporting goods stores and bike shops are also great sources of information. Many books have maps of local area hiking and biking trails. Larger cities may have recreational guides that list a variety of activities.

Use the form below to keep track of what you find:

NEW OPPORTUNITIES TO BE ACTIVE

Parks	Location	Comments
Recreation centers		

(continued)

(continued)

Activity clubs	Location	Comments
Other		

As you fill in this form, give careful thought to new physical activities or opportunities about which you'd like to learn more. Circle your top two and give them a try!

UP CLOSE & PERSONAL

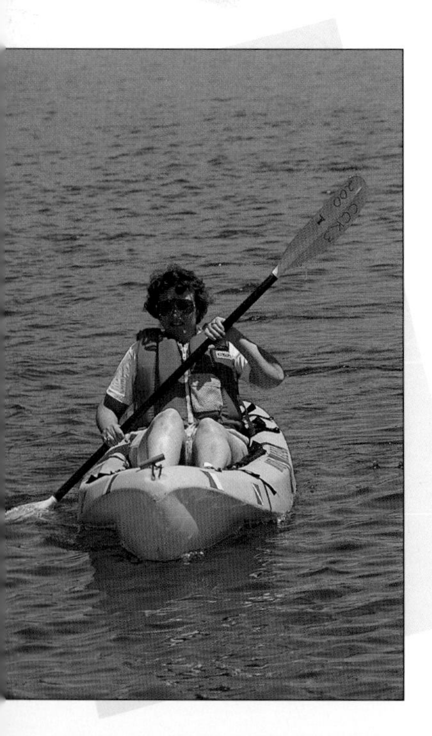

Cheryl had tried bicycling, hiking, and roller-blading, but none of them gave her much pleasure. Then one day, walking over the bridge in town, she noticed a group of people kayaking on the river. The small boats looked so graceful, and the activity of rowing seemed so peaceful, that Cheryl decided to give it a try. To her delight, she discovered through the parks and recreation department that her town had a rowing club. By joining, she could have access to kayaks or canoes at the wharf any time she wanted. All she had to do was pay a yearly membership and take three lessons in water safety.

Joining the rowing club came at just the right time in her life, shortly after her divorce and during a period when she was becoming depressed. Rowing, especially after work when the air was cool and the light was golden, helped her relax and restore her spirits. She made friends with the other rowers, who all had a welcome sense of camaraderie. Recently, Cheryl signed up for a vacation trip to Mexico, complete with a few days of kayaking off Baja. She's in the best physical shape of her life. Just as important, she's found a real passion.

Dance, Dance, Dance

Has it been ages since you put on your favorite music and kicked up your heels? Now might be the time to give dancing another try. Whether it's the Texas two-step or a stately waltz on the ballroom floor, dancing is a wonderful way to relax, enjoy yourself, and get some physical activity. It's great fun to dance with your kids or grandkids. Even dancing by yourself to the beat of your favorite songs can be a great way to unwind and get your heart rate up. Have some boring housework to do? Try putting on your favorite music and dancing while doing chores. Time will fly by and your house will be sparkling. If you want to get serious about dancing, check out the community listings for dance classes or dancing clubs.

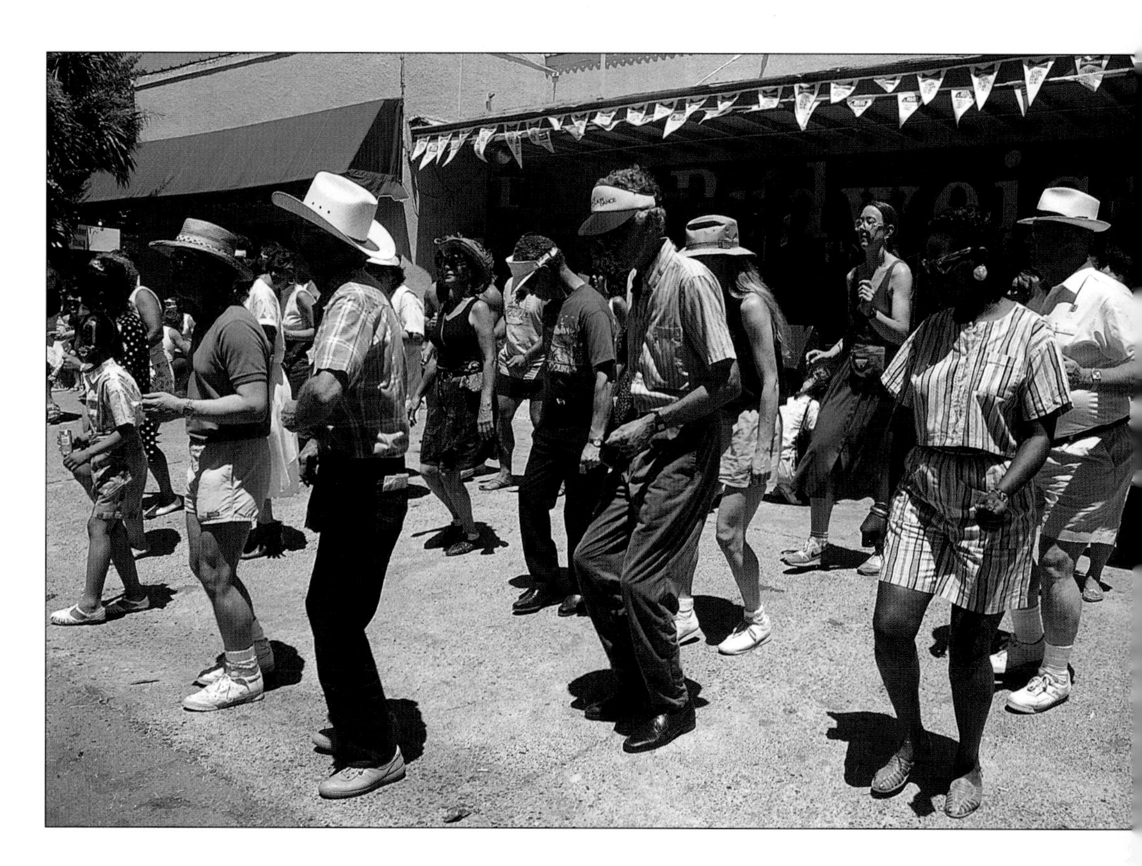

Dancing is a great way to be active!

Selecting Home Exercise Equipment

Activity groups and hiking trails aren't for everyone. Some people prefer to be active in the privacy of their homes. There are plenty of advantages to having home exercise equipment such as treadmills, stair climbers, or rowing machines. First is convenience—it's there whenever you feel the urge to get up and moving. At-home equipment is terrific for rainy days or days when it's too hot or cold to go outside. Just having equipment in the

DID YOU KNOW?

The convenience of having a treadmill at home could make it easy to be active and even lose a few extra pounds. In a study at the University of Pittsburgh,[17] researchers put 148 overweight women on a diet and assigned them to one of three five-day-a-week exercise programs. The first group was supposed to walk 40 minutes in a single session. The second and third groups divided their 40 minutes into 10-minute bouts. Women in the third group had an advantage: the researchers gave them treadmills to use at home.

After 18 months, the group exercising at home lost over 16 pounds (7.25 kg) while the first and second groups lost nearly 13 (5.9 kg) and 8 pounds (3.6 kg), respectively. Why? Home equipment such as a treadmill may be particularly appealing to people who are overweight and sensitive about how they look at the gym or walking around town. With home exercise equipment, you can work out whenever you want and wear whatever you want. Another important message from this study is that regardless of using long or short bouts, the more exercise you do, the more weight you lose (see following table).

Increased Physical Activity Leads to Greater Weight Loss

Minutes of exercise (per week)	Amount of weight loss in 18 months in lb (kg)
More than 200	28.8 (13.1)
150-200	18.7 (8.5)
Less than 150	7.7 (3.5)

Chapter Checklist

Before you move on to the next week's activities, make sure you

- Completed the New Opportunities to Be Active form
- Chose one or two new activities to try
- Considered options for renting or buying home exercise equipment

This week, you explored new opportunities to be active. Just by adding one or two alternatives to your list of fun things to do, you improve your odds of sticking with your plan to become an active person. Next week we'll look back at the strategies that have worked best for you. We'll even give you a chance to pat yourself on the back.

kayaking off Baja. She's in the best physical shape of her life. Just as important, she's found a real passion.

Dance, Dance, Dance

Has it been ages since you put on your favorite music and kicked up your heels? Now might be the time to give dancing another try. Whether it's the Texas two-step or a stately waltz on the ballroom floor, dancing is a wonderful way to relax, enjoy yourself, and get some physical activity. It's great fun to dance with your kids or grandkids. Even dancing by yourself to the beat of your favorite songs can be a great way to unwind and get your heart rate up. Have some boring housework to do? Try putting on your favorite music and dancing while doing chores. Time will fly by and your house will be sparkling. If you want to get serious about dancing, check out the community listings for dance classes or dancing clubs.

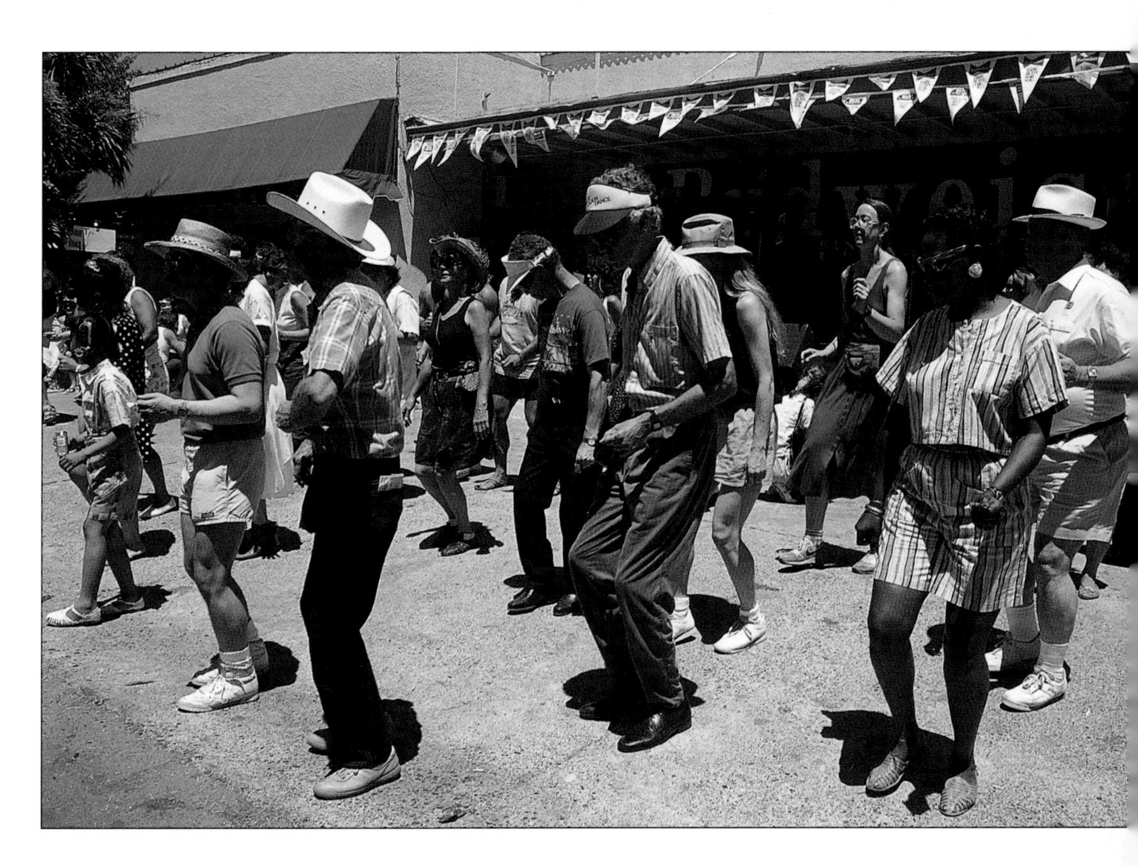

Dancing is a great way to be active!

Selecting Home Exercise Equipment

Activity groups and hiking trails aren't for everyone. Some people prefer to be active in the privacy of their homes. There are plenty of advantages to having home exercise equipment such as treadmills, stair climbers, or rowing machines. First is convenience—it's there whenever you feel the urge to get up and moving. At-home equipment is terrific for rainy days or days when it's too hot or cold to go outside. Just having equipment in the

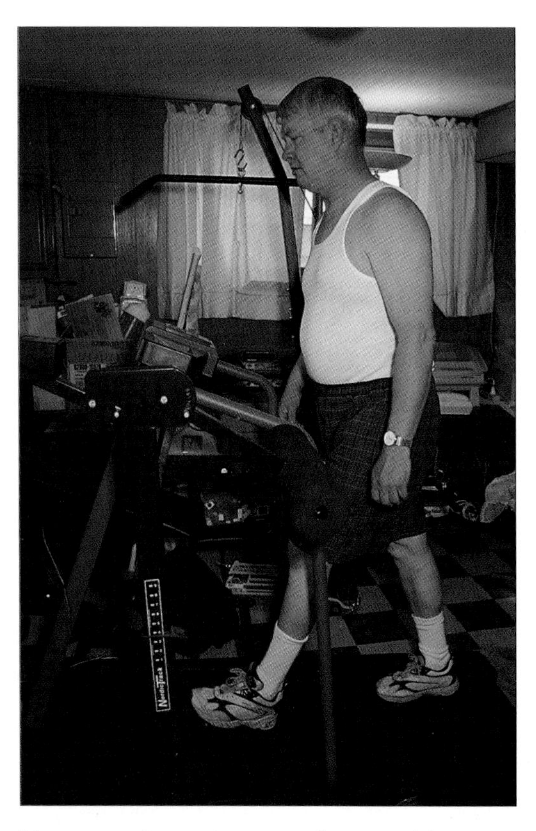

Home exercise equipment makes exercising convenient and carefree.

house is a reminder to be active. You can set up your treadmill or stair machine in front of a television and watch your favorite show. After all, you don't have to be a couch potato to enjoy a little TV time. You can also read or listen to music. Over time, buying your equipment can be cheaper than paying for a membership at a gym. What's more, several family members can use the exercise equipment. That's important because children who see their parents being active are likely to be active themselves.

Before you buy or rent equipment, consider a few potential drawbacks. If your activity interests change, you'll be stuck with a piece of equipment no one uses. Unless you have the space to set up the equipment and leave it in place, chances are it may spend more time in storage than in use. Equipment needs repair from time to time, which can be costly and inconvenient.

If the pros outweigh the cons for you, check out what local sporting stores offer. There are also stores that sell used exercise equipment, or look in the classified ads, where you can often find a great bargain. Be sure to try out equipment before you buy it. Here's a checklist of questions to ask to get the best products:

- Is the manufacturer reputable? How long have they been in business? What other products do they make?
- Does the equipment come with a warranty? What does it cover? Is there an additional charge for the warranty?
- Is electricity required to operate the equipment? (Motors and other electronic devices are prone to need repair.)
- Is the equipment adjustable for all sizes and fitness levels?
- How much does it cost?
- How much space is required to operate it?
- Is the equipment sturdy enough to last for several years?
- Are training instructions provided?
- Can you achieve your physical activity goals with this equipment?
- Is it safe?
- Do you think you would enjoy this equipment for a long time and use it regularly?

WEEK SEVENTEEN

Making Lasting Changes

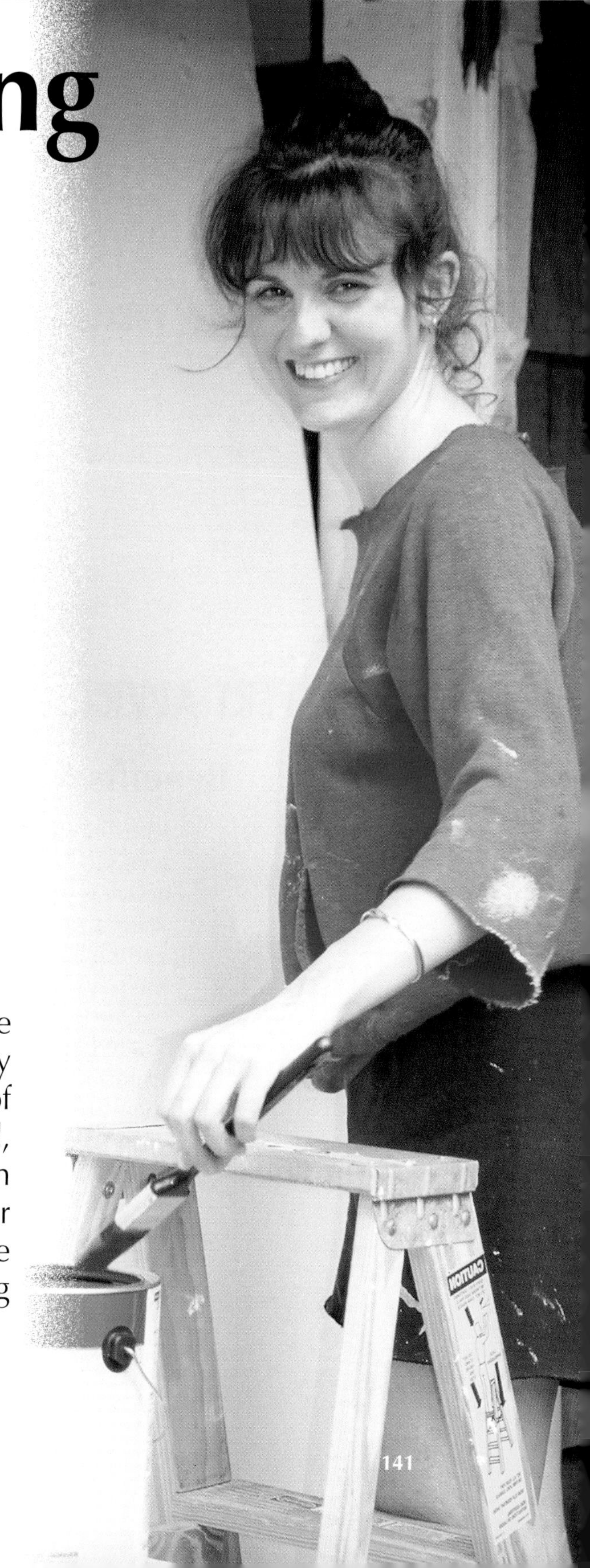

In This Chapter

- Celebrating your accomplishments
- Looking back at the activities you like best
- Trying new activities to renew your motivation

The aim of this book is to help you overcome obstacles and inspire you to become active every day—and for the rest of your life. In the end, of course, a single book, even the best in the world, can only help set you on the right path. Staying on course ultimately depends on you. In this chapter you'll have a chance to celebrate how far you've come and think about ways to make lasting changes.

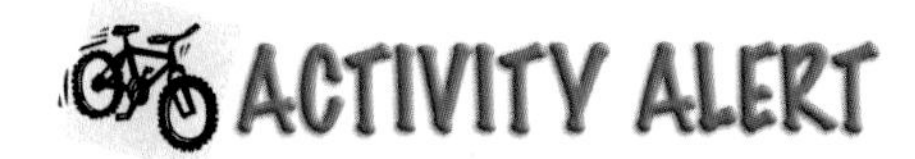

Positive Changes

Celebrations such as a birthday or a New Year's party offer a chance to think back over the time gone by and anticipate what lies ahead. Over the past several months you've worked hard at making and keeping a resolution to include activity in your daily life—hard enough that you deserve to celebrate. One way to do that is to think about what you have accomplished. Right now, before you go any further, jot down in the margin a few positive changes you've experienced along the way. Review them and list your top three here:

THREE REASONS TO CELEBRATE

1. ______________________________

2. ______________________________

3. ______________________________

EXPERT ADVICE

Benefits Keep Growing

More energy, greater self-confidence, lower blood pressure and cholesterol levels, a brighter outlook on life—whatever you've gained from becoming active is important. Stick with it, the evidence shows, and the benefits will keep adding up. Studies show that the longer you keep to your goal of getting 30 minutes or more of at least moderate-intensity activity, the bigger the payoff in health.

One benefit you may not have listed is as important as any of the others. We're talking about getting to know yourself better. For many people, the experience of making an important and lasting change in lifestyle gives them an insight into themselves. Someone who decides to spend a few hours each week doing something for a local charity, for instance, may be surprised to learn how much he or she enjoys working with children or older people. Someone who tries to quit smoking may be startled to discover how much hard work and willpower it takes to quit for good. Along the way he or she may discover unexpected reserves of personal strength and commitment.

Along the way in our program, chances are good you've learned some things about yourself. Not all of them have to be positive. There's nothing wrong with discovering that you have to push yourself hard to get up and be active, or that you don't like riding a bicycle. We hope some things you've learned about yourself have given you new self-confidence.

ACTIVITY ALERT

What Have You Learned?

Take a moment to think about the past few months. What strengths and weaknesses have you seen in yourself as you've tried to change your lifestyle? Write down a few of the most important insights. Getting to know yourself will help you get past the biggest hurdle that lies ahead: making a real and lasting change in your lifestyle.

THREE THINGS I'VE LEARNED ABOUT MYSELF

1. ____________________

2. ____________________

3. ____________________

UP CLOSE & PERSONAL

When Hye-Suk joined Project *Active*, he had tried and failed in his efforts to shape up and slim down so often that he'd begun to think of himself as a failure. No sooner would he make a resolution to go on a diet or begin to exercise than a voice in his head would say, "You've never succeeded before. What makes you think you'll do it this time?"

Early in the program, thinking about obstacles that got in his way, Hye-Suk became aware of the voice in his head. For the first time he realized that the discouraging voice was there no matter what he attempted to do. Becoming aware of the negative messages in his head was a revelation. Learning to counter those negative messages with positive ones gave Hye-Suk an unexpected sense of possibility. "I can do it if I really want to," he'd tell himself. "Of course people have setbacks," he'd remind himself.

Hye-Suk found himself not only sticking with his goal of activity but also enjoying every minute of it. Something else even more important than reaching his goal happened: Hye-Suk banished the negative and demoralizing voice in his head. Now, whenever it pops up, he simply turns "can't" into "can." He's begun to think about himself and his life with confidence and enthusiasm.

I can't walk any further
I've discovered so many new things on my walking route. I'm glad I'm out here.

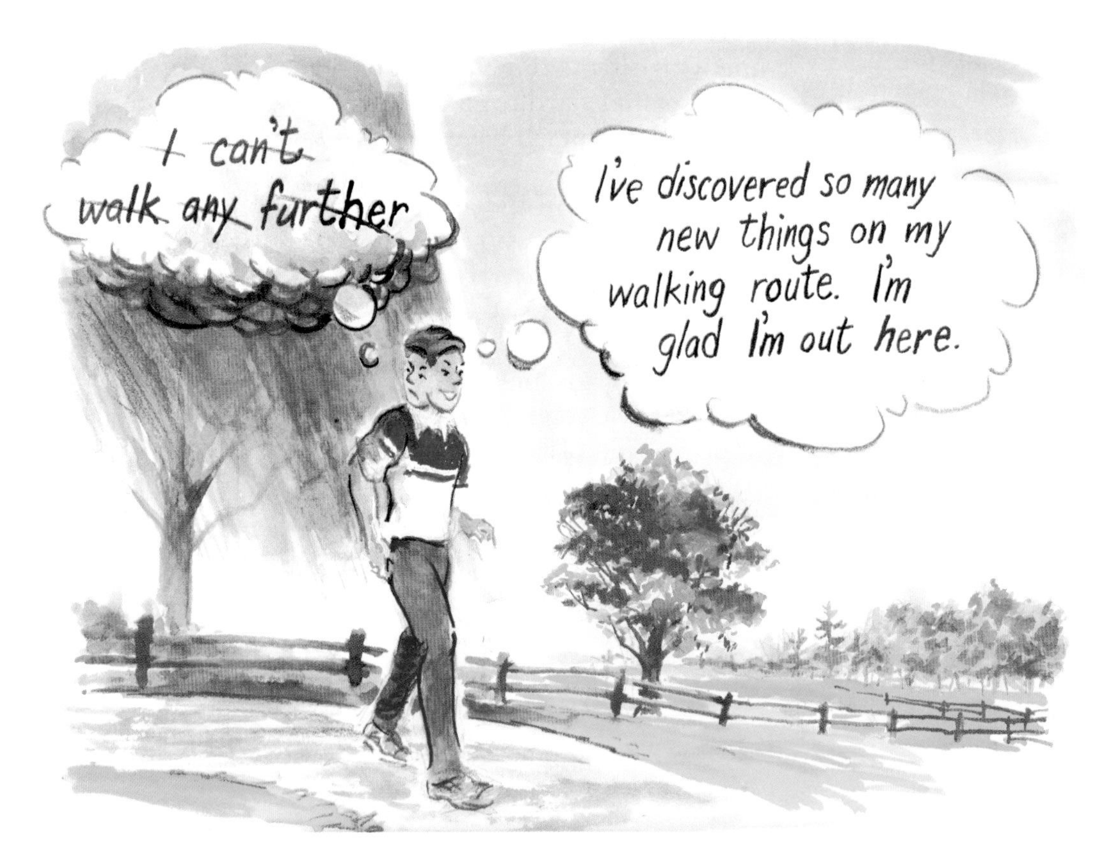

EXPERT ADVICE

What's *Your* Secret for Success?

Magazines are brimming with stories that offer the secrets to success, whether it's successful weight loss, ageless beauty, or financial independence. There is no one secret to success of any kind. Success takes many steps. When it comes to shaping up with an active lifestyle, success means doing something active every day.

Take a minute to think about what has worked best for you. Perhaps it was keeping track of how you spent your time each day. Maybe you began to make real strides when you started using a step counter. Some people make a big change after they understand the obstacles that get in their way. Others take a giant step forward when they learn simple ways to problem solve.

The people in Project *Active* and our other studies tried many activities and strategies. After giving them a fair try, they found some worked better than others. Here are a few examples:

- Nancy found that her love of nature, specifically walking on trails through the woods near her home, kept her motivated through rain or shine, hot or cold. When she had foot surgery, she had to give up walking for a while. It wasn't long before she felt sluggish, grouchy, and sorry for herself. After two months of inactivity, getting started wasn't easy. She began by walking in the local pool to get back in shape.

Fortunately, spring was just beginning to burst out. The lure of daffodils coming up and trees beginning to leaf out was enough to get her back to her daily schedule of walking half an hour after work.

- For Charisse, variety was the key to success. Before, when she joined a gym, she quickly tired of the stair machines and treadmills and stopped going altogether. Now she's learned to love spinning, box aerobics, bicycling, and a brisk walk through the neighborhood. She and her fiancé have even begun participating in fun runs together.
- Miguel's secret to success can be described in one word: bicycling. He hadn't pedaled a bike since he was in high school, more years ago than he wanted to count. When a friend suggested going on a short ride into the country, he decided to give it a try. It had been years since he'd had so much fun. From that day on, he scheduled at least three short rides around the neighborhood after work each week and one longer ride during the weekends. Now he's training for a 50K ride. "Frankly, I never would have gotten this far if I hadn't found something I loved to do—something that made it worthwhile," he admits.

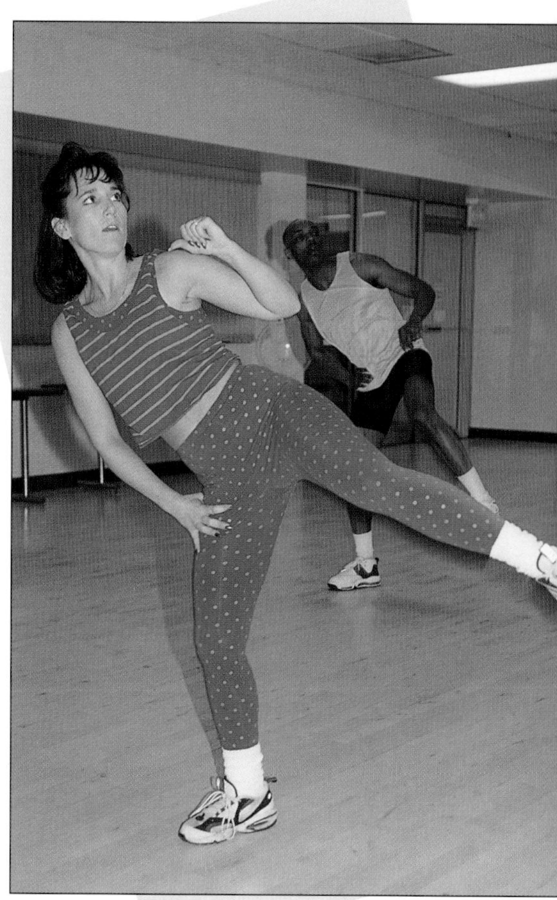

One key to staying active is finding an activity that you enjoy.

ACTIVITY ALERT

What Works for You?

Think back over the past few months, and make a list of what has worked best for you. Include the activities you've enjoyed the most, and think about the strategies that have worked well, such as time management or overcoming obstacles. If you haven't achieved all your goals, don't be discouraged. Although it is important to learn what works, some of us progress by first learning what doesn't work. If you haven't been able to stay motivated, for instance, think about what you've tried that hasn't worked, then write down a few alternatives you think might help your motivation.

(continued)

(continued)

KEYS TO MY SUCCESS

1. ______________________________

2. ______________________________

3. ______________________________

4. ______________________________

5. ______________________________

6. ______________________________

Renewing Your Motivation

One of the best ways to stay motivated is to get together with other people to share ideas and strategies for adding fun activities to your daily routine. Chances are you'll learn something you never thought about before. We've learned some surprising things from participants in Project *Active* when we asked them to bring in items that represented the physical activity they liked to do.

For example, one participant brought a paperback book. This was puzzling until she explained that when she first tried to become active, she always felt as if she'd rather curl up with a good book. As she thought about her habits and where to fit in activity, she decided to use her love of reading as her reward for activity well done. She was able to discipline herself to walk before reading. By the end of the program she was walking three miles a day and had read almost 100 books.

Another participant built his activity around his children. Setting a good example for them was his main motive for increasing his activity in the first place, he explained. So the more unusual and zany the activity, the more fun he and his kids had. They roller-bladed, juggled, and learned to ride a unicycle. Of course, not everyone can or wants to learn circus tricks to stay active, but the idea of playing with your kids or grandchildren can be a rewarding way to add activity to family life.

There are other ways to keep inspired. For starters, look back over the list of activities you scouted out in your community (week 16). Choose one or two new ones you might like to try. Over the next couple weeks, keep a sharp eye out for what other people are doing to stay active. If someone you admire at work or in the neighborhood has found a way to keep motivated, ask about his or her secret.

Chapter Checklist

Before you move on to the next week's activities, make sure you

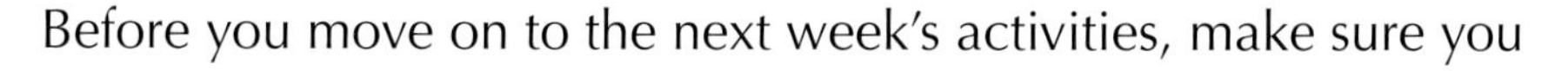

- Listed your top three reasons to celebrate your progress so far
- Listed three important things you've learned about yourself
- Identified strategies that have helped you succeed

Change is a process of getting to know yourself. Gaining insight into what motivates you is an important part of the progress you're making. In the next chapter, we'll explore a few ways to add activities to your weekly schedule. You'll also have a chance to make a new set of short-term and long-term goals.

WEEK **EIGHTEEN**

Becoming a Hunter-Gatherer

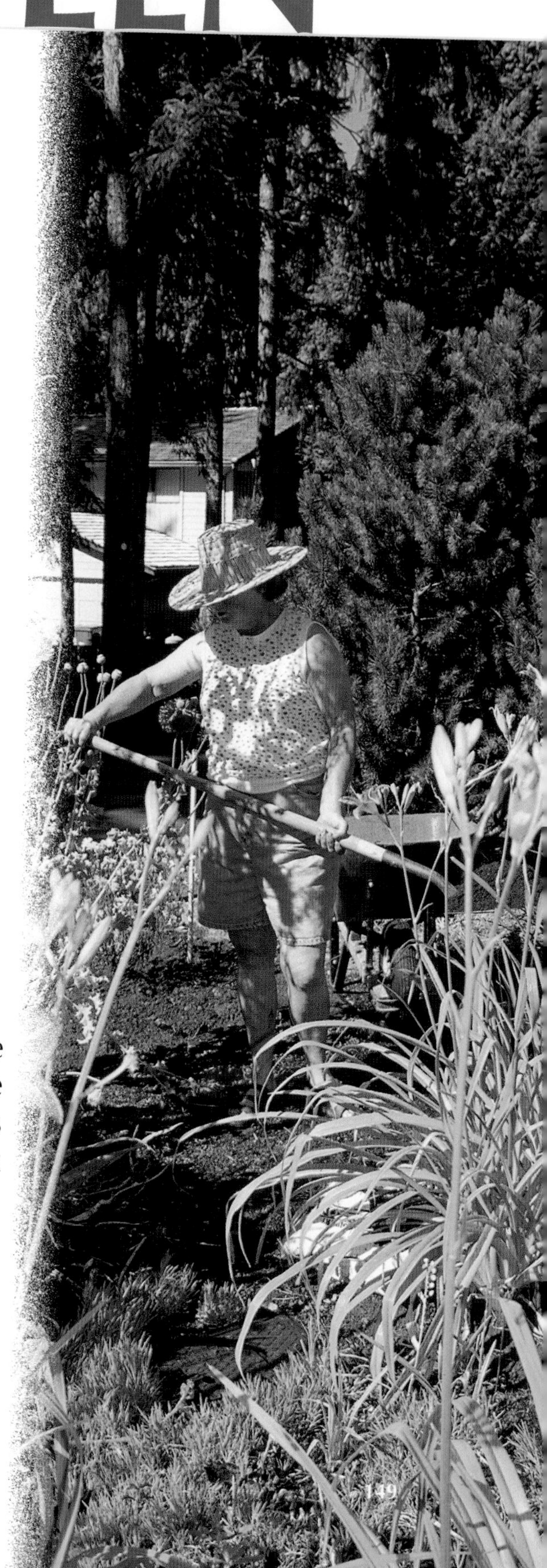

In This Chapter

- Adding a little extra activity to your weekly schedule
- Setting new goals to stay motivated
- Taking another look at the causes of overweight and obesity

With so many labor-saving inventions taking the burden off us, it's no surprise so many people are becoming sedentary. The problem is, our bodies were built to be active. In this chapter we'll look at a few simple ways to get back to our roots.

How Times Have Changed

If someone from the 1850s could travel through time to the present, he or she would be astonished. Machines have taken over many back-breaking jobs that were an essential part of life. Back then, doing housework was a physically demanding job. Making roads, building houses, and growing crops all required hours of physical labor.

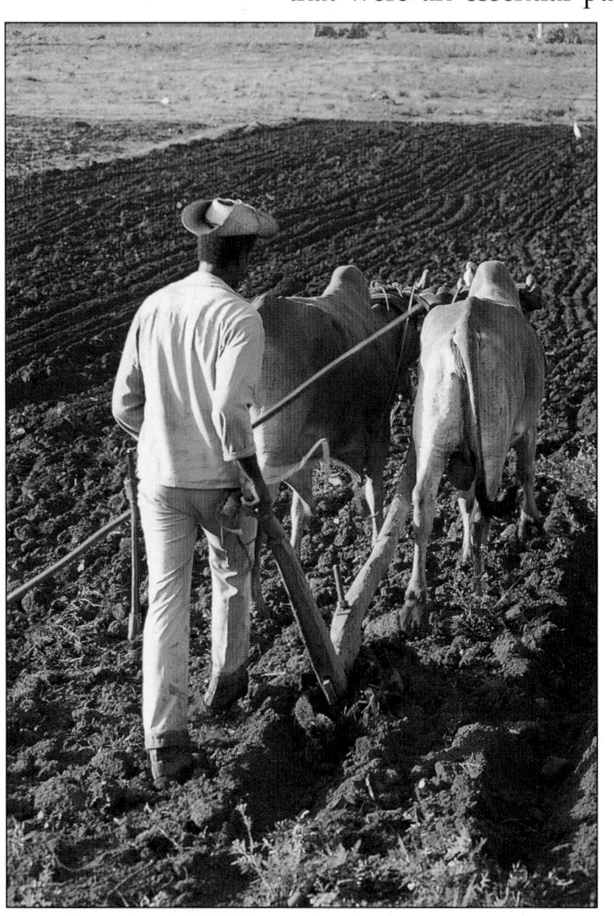

This Cuban farmer reaps the benefits of his physical labor.

In fact, our bodies were designed for strenuous activity. We once lived as hunter-gatherers, humans who spent much of the day moving about and working hard to get enough to eat. Our bodies require physical activity to be healthy. Back in Fred and Wilma Flintstone's time, we also had to adapt to periods when food was scarce. Hence, our bodies found ways to store excess calories as body fat when food was plentiful so that we'd have a source of energy when food became scarce.

Problem is, there's not much left to do that demands strenuous activity. On top of that, we've created a world of unprecedented plenty, with a greater variety of foods than many people dreamed of in previous generations.

Life may be easier (and more delicious), but we're paying the price in obesity, heart disease, and other chronic diseases.

Of course, we can't go back to being hunter-gatherers. But to be healthy, we must find ways to resist the sedentary pressures of today's modern world.

? DID YOU KNOW?

For years, scientists funded by the National Institutes of Health have been studying the Pima Indians in Arizona, in hopes of helping them fight a dangerous epidemic. By now, you know that too many Americans are overweight or obese, but the Pimas in the United States suffer an extraordinarily high incidence of obesity. As many as 75 percent are obese. Partly as a result, many suffer from diabetes.

Yet when scientists traveled to a remote part of Mexico where the Pimas' ancestors still live much the way they have for thousands of years, they discovered something surprising. The Pimas who tilled the land and carried water by hand were lean and remarkably healthy. Researchers found virtually no diabetes or obesity among the Mexican Pimas.

Why, then, are the Pima Indians in the United States plagued by obesity? First, these Pimas got significantly less physical activity than the Pimas in

Mexico.[18] Researchers also suspect that the Pimas adapted to their harsh environment by evolving to make every calorie of energy they ate go as far as it could. Those most likely to survive were those who had what scientists have called a thrifty gene. When food was scarce this gene kept people alive.

Unfortunately in the United States, where food is plentiful and machines do the hard work, a thrifty gene seems to be dangerous. It predisposes people to obesity and all the health problems that come with it.

The Pima Indians of Arizona and Mexico illustrate a problem many of us face. Our bodies were built for a different environment. In our current world, we have to work hard not to gain weight. All of us would be healthier if we could add more physical activity into our lives than we currently do.

EXPERT ADVICE

Striving for Increased Benefits

If you've stuck with us this far, chances are you're meeting the official public health guidelines for physical activity—to accumulate 30 minutes or more of moderate-intensity activity on most, preferably all, days of the week.

That's great, especially if you started out completely sedentary. As the figure below shows, the biggest health gains are whenever you go from being sedentary to meeting the recommended level. But while you're patting yourself on your back, remember this: doing a little bit more than the recommended level would mean even bigger benefits than you are getting now. Our work at The Cooper Institute—in fact, most studies of exercise and health—show that the benefits of activity are dose dependent. That's jargon for a simple idea: the more you do, the more benefits you'll get.

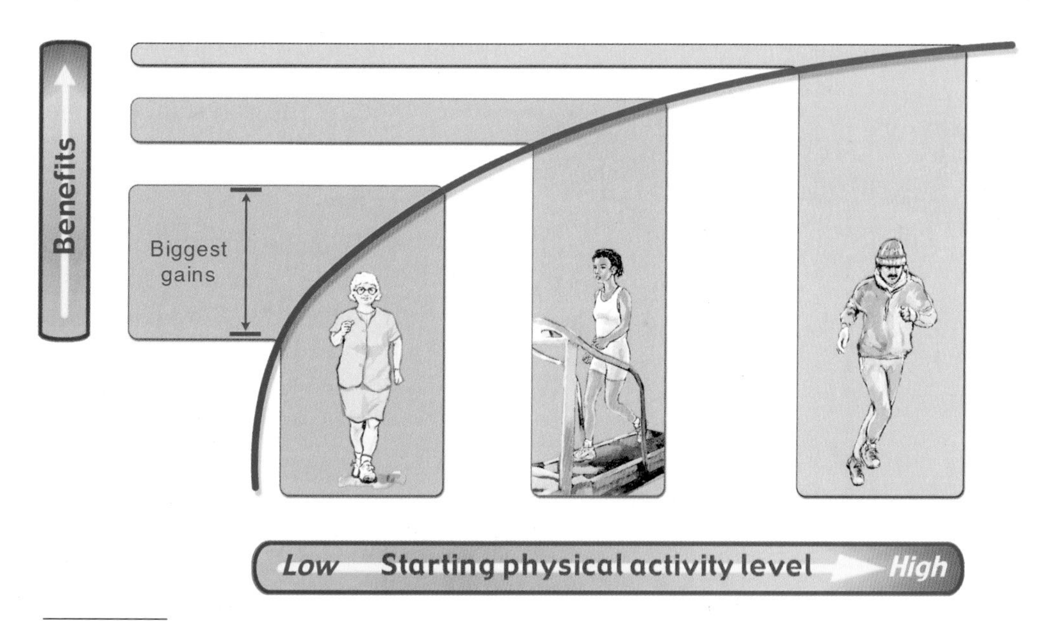

Your greatest health gains will occur when you first start exercising, going from a sedentary lifestyle to the recommended activity level; you will continue reaping benefits with even more exercise.
Adapted, by permission, from R.R. Pate, M. Pratt, S.N. Blair, et al., 1995, "Physical activity and public health," *JAMA* 273 (5): 402-407.

ACTIVITY ALERT

A Week's Worth of Activities

So, here they are: a week's worth of ways to increase your activity. Some may already be part of your lifestyle. Others may be new. Your mission is to commit yourself to doing each one. Depending on your schedule, you may need to trade one day's activities for another. No problem. Mark each activity on your daily calendar.

Sunday

Add an extra quarter mile (.4 km) to your walk or pick up the pace of whatever activity you do. Building endurance will increase your staying power for all your activities.

Monday

For every trip you take during the day, park your car as far away from your destination as possible. You may do away with the stress of finding a close parking space, and you'll add a useful way to expend energy. If you don't drive, get off the bus a stop or two earlier than your destination.

Tuesday

Instead of dessert at lunch, take a walk. Invite a friend to come along.

Wednesday

Find a mall close to work or home and go buy that thingamajig you keep forgetting. While you're at it, tally up an extra 15 minutes of brisk walking.

Thursday

While the kids are at soccer practice (or baseball, hockey, football, marching band, or dance), walk around the field a few times or take a brisk walk through the neighborhood. Don't have kids who play sports? You can still find a field or park to walk around.

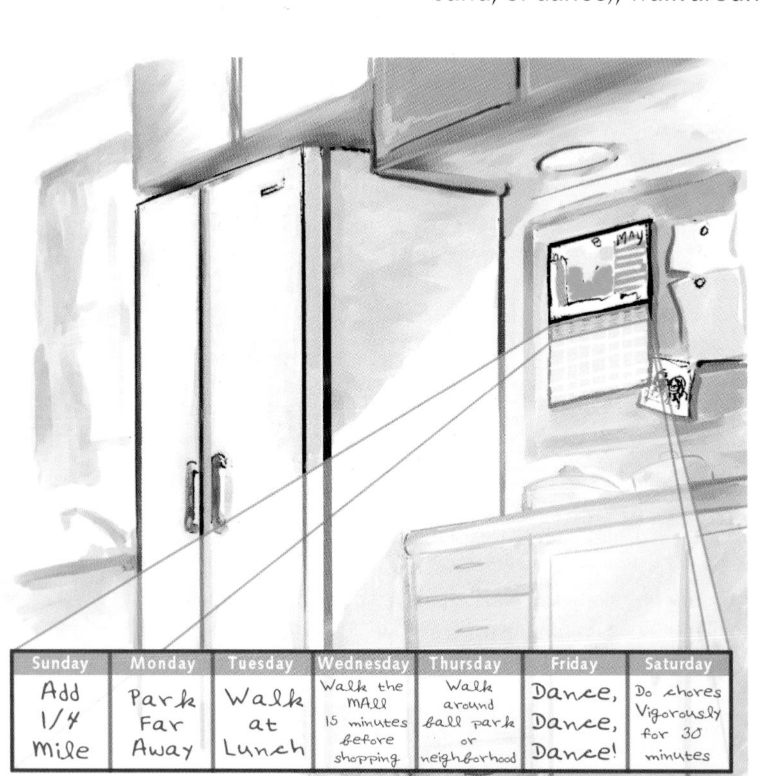

Friday

Get out the drums! Put on the music! It's time to dance! Celebrate a successful week of hunter-gathering by grooving to whatever music you enjoy, alone or with someone you love. If you have a favorite local dance club, go for it. If not, boogie across the living room floor.

Saturday

Chores, chores, chores—it's time to get out there and catch up on active jobs such as weeding in the garden, mowing the lawn (no riding mowers, please), doing home repairs, or doing vigorous housework such as mopping the floor. Put in at least 30 minutes.▌

UP CLOSE & PERSONAL

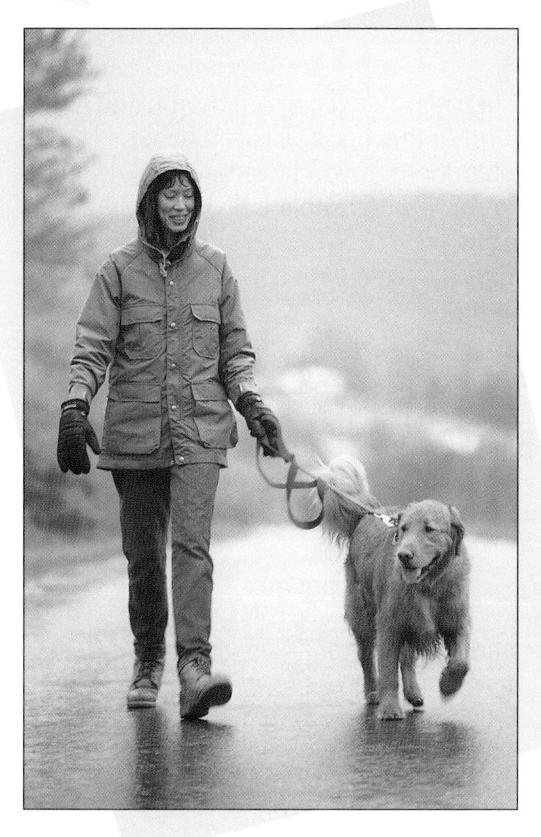

For years Paula had wanted a dog. Unfortunately the apartment she lived in didn't allow pets. "If only I had a dog who insisted on a walk," she told herself, "I'd be more active."

Then one day, taking a new route on her evening walk, she happened by a local school yard, where dog owners were allowed to have their pets play off the leash. Suddenly Paula had an idea. A few days later she put up signs for a dog-walking service.

It didn't take long for the phone to begin ringing. Within a month she had a regular clientele. Because she worked at home as a freelance illustrator, she was able to take time in the morning, over lunch, or in the evening to run her second business. One owner hired her to walk his collie over the noon hour, because he often worked long hours and didn't get home until late. Another dog owner, who traveled for work, hired Paula to look after her dog a few days a week while she was on the road.

Paula loved every minute of it. Before long she was walking at least an hour a day, often more. Thanks to a clever idea, she was able to combine physical activity with a new part-time job. As if that wasn't enough, she finally had a dog, or rather, a dozen dogs in her life.

WEIGHING IN

Are some people born to be overweight? For years researchers have recognized that obesity and overweight run in families. A child born to overweight parents is more likely to be overweight than a child born to parents who are not obese.

Researchers don't fully understand what inherited characteristics lead people to be more likely to gain weight. Some experts think the problem may lie in faulty satiety signals, the messages that go from stomach to brain to say, "enough already, I'm full." Other researchers think we may have different metabolic set points, which determine how much body fat we have. There may be other reasons.

Most likely, a combination of inherited characteristics predispose certain people to put on too much weight. Remember that word predispose. No one is *fated* to be fat. Certainly, obesity is also determined by the world we live in and the way we live in it. In fact, many experts think that environment may play a much bigger role than heredity.

The good news is that you can manage to achieve a healthy weight for your body type, but it means controlling your environment. For most people, that involves keeping a close eye on diet and being as active as possible every day.

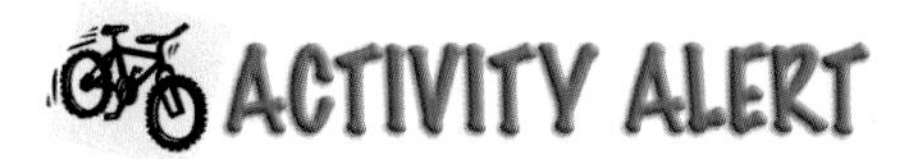

Pushing Harder

All you have to do is feel the number of pages between your thumb and finger to know you're getting close to the end of this book. That's why we've been encouraging you to push just a little harder than you have been. We want to make sure that when the book is done you'll stick with all the healthy changes you've made.

Many people find it easier to reach a goal if they put it in writing. So get out your pen or pencil—it's commitment time.

MY PLAN TO PUSH A LITTLE HARDER

1. Do you plan to increase or maintain your current activity level? (Circle one.)

   Increase   Maintain

2. If you are planning to increase activity level, circle the things you plan to increase:

   Frequency   Types of activities

   Amount of time (duration)   Intensity

3. Now list the strategies you will use to put your plan into action. Remember to be specific. (Check all that apply.)

   ☐ Set new short-term goal(s):

   ____

   ____

   ☐ Reward myself with ____________ for meeting my short-term goal.

   ☐ Set new long-term goal(s):

   ____

   ____

   ☐ Reward myself with ____________ for meeting my long-term goal.

❐ Self-monitor using either a step counter or by keeping track of minutes. (Circle one.)

Step counter   Minutes

❐ Enlist my support troops:

____

____

❐ Try a new activity:

____

____

❐ Plan for high-risk situations:

____

____

NEED A BOOST?

The more active you are, the easier it becomes to think of yourself as an active person and the easier it is to stick with the exercise habit. Still, problems can come along that threaten to knock you off track. A busy period at work, a family crisis, an illness, or a period when you feel blah all can get in your way. If you need a little push now and then, here are a few simple ways to motivate yourself:

- Ask someone close to you to help you problem solve the issues that are holding you back.
- Keep track of your plans, goals, and activities. Keeping an activity log is a powerful motivator.
- Push yourself to try one or two new activities.
- Explore your home, neighborhood, or work environments to discover new places and ways to be active.
- Each night before you go to bed, write in your calendar when and how you are going to fit in activity the next day.
- Go back to an earlier chapter if you feel the need for a refresher course.

Chapter Checklist

Before you move on to the next week's activities, make sure you

- [ ] Completed a week's worth of ways to increase your activity
- [ ] Made a plan to push yourself a little harder in the weeks to come

As you'll discover, many strategies you used to get yourself moving in the first place can help you push yourself a little harder now. The more you do, the more benefits you'll get from an active lifestyle. Of course, you'll encounter road bumps now and then. Who doesn't? In the coming week we'll take another look at overcoming obstacles that can get in the way.

WEEK NINETEEN

Positive Planning

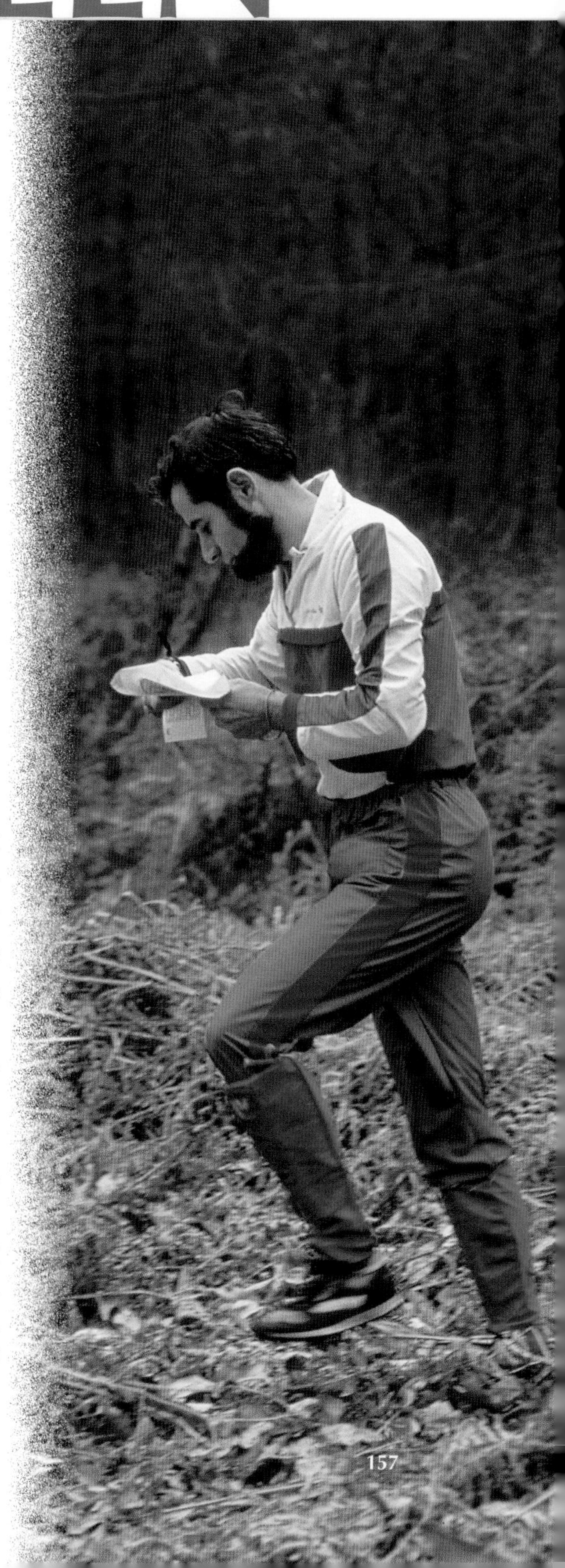

In This Chapter

- Turning negative messages into a positive attitude
- Preparing for situations that can throw you off track
- Planning to increase your activity

By now, we hope that you've begun to think about yourself and your life differently. You've convinced yourself that you can plan and follow through on a goal to increase your activity. Like many people in our programs, you may have switched from thinking of yourself as a couch potato to seeing yourself as an active person who enjoys getting up and *doing* something.

Even the most committed, active-minded people, however, face times when it's not easy to stick to their resolutions. Just by living our lives, we all encounter new barriers that we need to get around to keep activity a top priority. In this chapter we'll remind you of strategies to keep your plans flexible so you can steer clear of trouble and stay on track.

Making It Last

One important advantage of a lifestyle approach to activity is that it is adaptable. You don't have to worry about finding a gym nearby or shaping your schedule around workout hours. You don't even have to work up a hard sweat.

By now you know that many types of physical activity count as exercise, from walking and yard work to climbing stairs and playing volleyball with the kids. As long as physical activity is at least moderate intensity, it will improve your fitness and other measures of good health. The more you do the more you'll benefit.

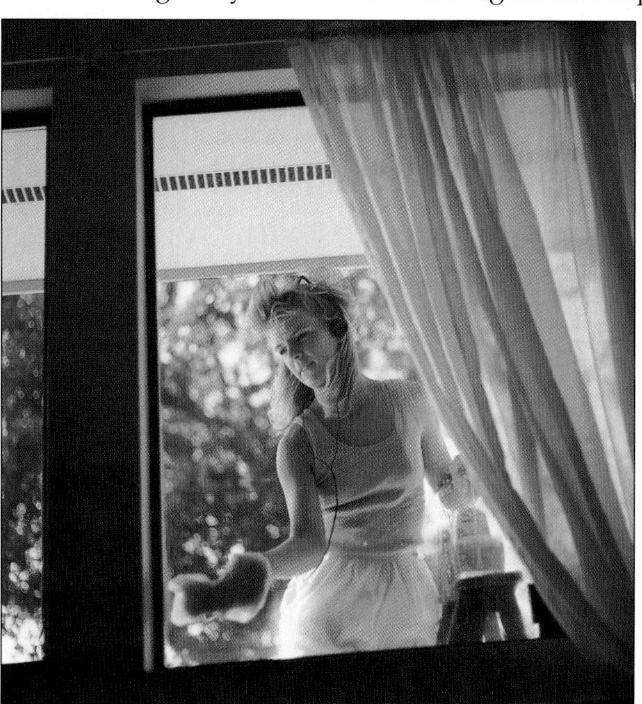

Staying fit doesn't have to mean going to the gym or changing your daily schedule.

You've also learned along the way that you can fit activity into your daily life no matter how crowded or hectic your schedule is. Whether you're a single parent with small children, a busy professional with many demands, both a single parent and a busy professional, or somewhere in between, you have time to be active if you plan for it.

We also hope you've realized that you need to expend energy to feel invigorated and healthy. Being active doesn't need to be hard work. It's a natural part of a healthy life. It can even be one of the most pleasurable parts of life.

EXPERT ADVICE

Your goal now is to maintain the physical activity habit you've been working so hard to establish. What will it take? Here are the keys:

1. **Good planning**

Whether you want to fit in a five-minute walk or a five-mile (8 km) hike, the key to making it happen is effective planning. We know from our studies that the people who get in the habit of setting aside time for physical activity are far more likely to remain active over the long run than those who don't plan ahead.

2. Flexibility

Remember, the path to making a lifelong change isn't always smooth. If you miss your planned activity for one day, be sure to make a plan for the following day, even if it's a five-minute walk. If you are injured, try an alternative activity if you can. If you're sick, wait until you're feeling better and gradually get back to your routine. If there's a problem at home or work, give it the priority it deserves, and resolve to get back to your activities as soon as you can. Set short-term and long-term goals. Find ways around new barriers through problem solving. Remind yourself of all the benefits you've gotten, or hope to get, from staying active.

3. Positive attitude

Nothing is more discouraging than a voice in your head that says, "I can't." Negative thinking and all-or-nothing thinking are two of the biggest obstacles many people face. A positive attitude and encouraging mental messages, on the other hand, can go a long way toward helping people to get past rocky times and stick to their commitment.

ACTIVITY ALERT

What Do You Think?

We've said it before, but it bears repeating: how you think has an impact on your success or failure. Do you feel discouraged when you've missed a few days of activity? Do you still hear a negative voice in your head? Now's the time to erase negative messages and replace them with words of encouragement.

1. Identify the negative thought. Too many people let negative thoughts get to them—as soon as they realize they've lapsed, they collapse. Typical negative thoughts are "I'm a failure," "I'll never be able to stick with my plan," or "I've failed before and I'll probably fail again."

2. Decide whether the thought is right or wrong. (*Hint:* It's usually wrong.) Of course, we want you to take your plan for activity seriously. It's reasonable to be concerned if you've gotten off track for a few weeks in a row. However, no one is a failure because they don't meet their plan one day, a week, or even longer. That's an example of destructive all-or-nothing thinking.

My Plan
to get back on track
I Can do it!
-Walk 15 minutes before work
-Ask Jared to go Cycling with me on Saturdays
-Make a list of new activities to try

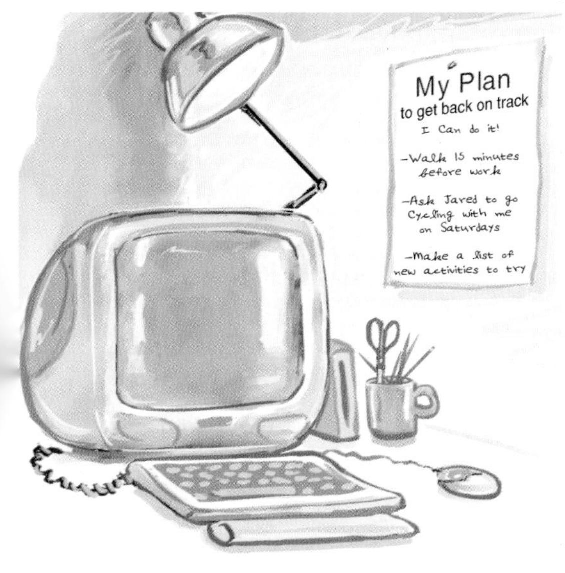

3. Counter the negative thought with a more accurate, reasonable, and positive response. If you find yourself thinking, "I haven't stuck with it, and I'm never going to be able to do it," instead, tell yourself, "I'm having a setback, but it doesn't have to be permanent. I'm still committed to being active and I know I can do it. I've worked through problems before and I can do it again." Remind yourself of ways you have done this by reviewing previous weeks in the book.

4. Make a specific plan. For instance, decide right now to put a short walk back into your routine each day to get yourself back on track again.

UP CLOSE & PERSONAL

By the end of participating in our lifestyle program, James had been through so many ups and downs he might as well have been on a roller coaster.

At the beginning, he surpassed his expectations, quickly racking up at least 30 minutes of brisk walking every day. Then came a badly sprained knee from an accident at work, which kept him on crutches for almost one week and out of commission for three. No sooner was he back to walking 30 minutes a day than there was a death in the family. Almost a month passed before his life returned to normal after that. He was proud of himself for quickly returning to his activity routine. Then a busy stretch at work forced him to miss doing his planned activities.

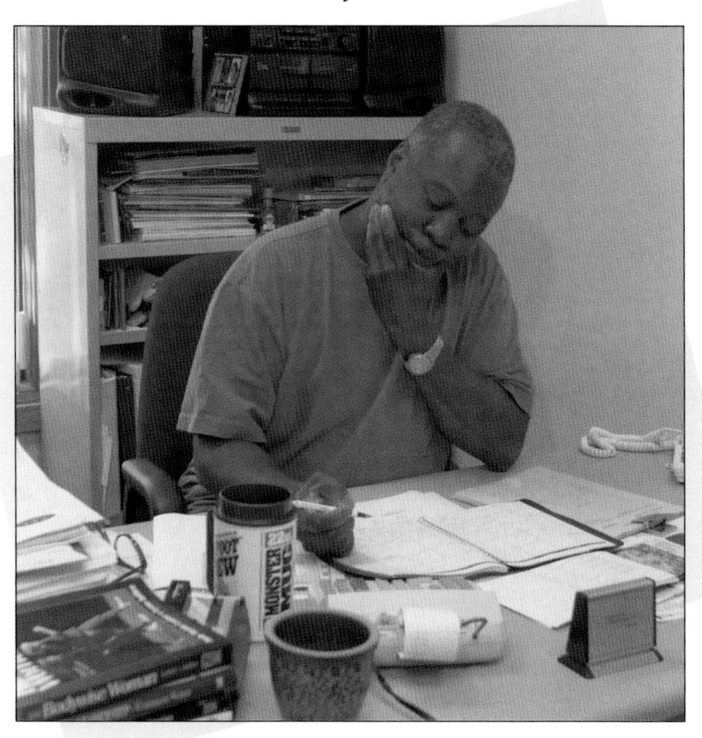

After that, James began to think the whole thing wasn't worth the trouble. After feeling so confident, he began to say to himself, "This is never going to work."

One day, hearing that voice in his head, he stopped and took stock. First, he told himself, he wasn't a quitter. He knew from experience that if he could get hold of the problem, he could solve it. As he often did when difficulties arose at work, he sat down, wrote out the problem, and listed ideas for solutions. He began to have insights into his way of thinking and acting.

For starters, he realized that he would always have to set goals for himself and plan to be active. At least for now, it wasn't something that came naturally to him. Thinking over the past few months, he also realized how important planning was for him. He tended to lose sight of his priorities when he found himself without a plan.

Finally, he began to understand how important it was for him to remind himself of the benefits of being active. He felt better, his blood pressure and cholesterol had fallen, and he felt less stressed-out when he stuck to his routine of walking. Somehow, he told himself, he had to keep those benefits in mind when things got rocky.

James made a few simple changes. He clipped out an advertising slogan—"No Excuses"—and put it on the refrigerator at home. He began writing his activity plan onto his work schedule, making sure that nothing got in the way. Every time he finished doing something he'd planned—walking, riding a bike, or working in the yard—he would stop, take a deep breath, notice the pleasant tiredness in his legs and arms, and appreciate how good it felt to be doing something good for himself.

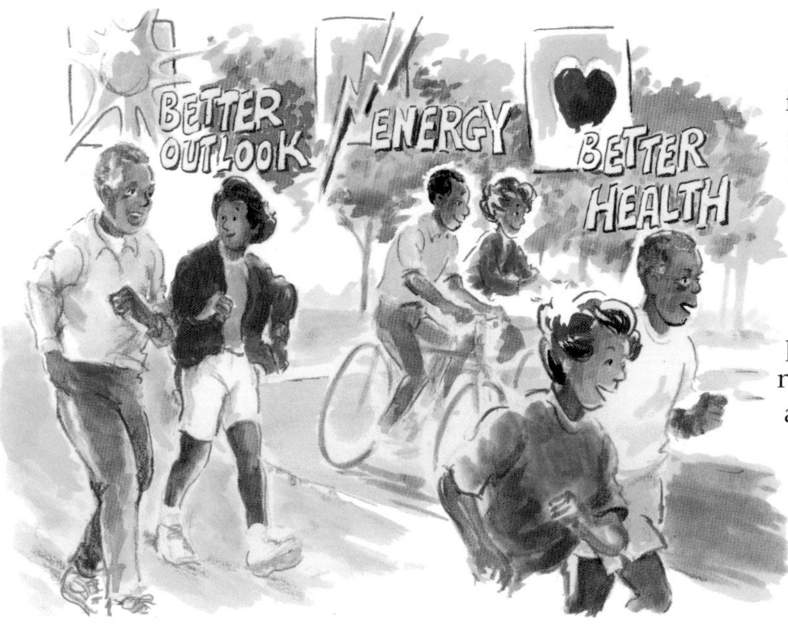

The longer you stick with your program for activity, the easier it will become. Like many participants in our studies, you may begin to think of yourself as an active person—someone for whom walking, cycling, hiking, and other activities comes naturally.

That doesn't mean you won't have to plan ahead or set goals for yourself. Planning and goal setting will help you move ahead and overcome obstacles that are sure to appear from time to time.

Planning and goal setting help you reap the benefits of physical activity.

ACTIVITY ALERT

Put It In Writing

It's a good idea to revisit your plans and goals regularly to focus on where you are and where you hope to go. Here's an opportunity to review and update your plans for activity. Of course, we couldn't be happier if you decide to add a bit more to your weekly routine. But even if you decide you're doing as much activity as you can manage right now, here's a pat on the back. As the benefits of an active lifestyle add up—increased energy, a bright outlook, good health—chances are you'll want to plan more activity than you have been doing.

Take a few minutes to answer the following questions and fine-tune your plan. We have a good reason to ask you to put it in writing. A plan is a contract you make with yourself. If it's in writing, chances are good you'll take it seriously.

FINE-TUNING YOUR PLAN

1. How often do you include physical activity in your daily schedule? (Circle one.)

   0 times a week   1-2 times a week
   3-4 times a week   5-7 times a week

2. If your plan includes physical activity 5 to 7 days a week, congratulations, and keep up the good work. If you haven't reached your goal yet, remember that every step forward is important. Do you think you're ready to plan more activity? (Circle one.)

   Yes   No

(continued)

(continued)

3. If yes, make a specific plan using the following schedule.

Day (Circle one or more)	**Activity** (Specify how many minutes or steps)
Monday	______________________
Tuesday	______________________
Wednesday	______________________
Thursday	______________________
Friday	______________________
Saturday	______________________
Sunday	______________________

ACTIVITY ALERT

Troubleshooting Revisited

Not quite meeting your goals? There may be an easy way around the problem. Here's an opportunity to do some constructive troubleshooting.

MY PLANS FOR TROUBLESHOOTING

1. First, think about the barriers in your way. If you aren't managing to meet your plan, why not? List the biggest obstacles.

   a. ______________________

   b. ______________________

   c. ______________________

2. Do you still find yourself discouraged by negative thoughts? (Circle one.)

   Never Rarely Sometimes Always

3. If so, what are they? List the negative messages that get in your way. Then think about ways to counter them and write your positive response.

Negative thought	**Positive response**
a.____________________	____________________________
b.____________________	____________________________
c.____________________	____________________________

4. Do you feel confident that you can maintain your program of physical activity no matter what problems arise? (Circle one.)

   Almost always Sometimes Rarely Almost never

5. If you answered "rarely" or "almost never," think about steps you can take to feel more confident than you do now. One way is to set more realistic short- and long-term goals. Create a specific plan and write it down.

____

____

____

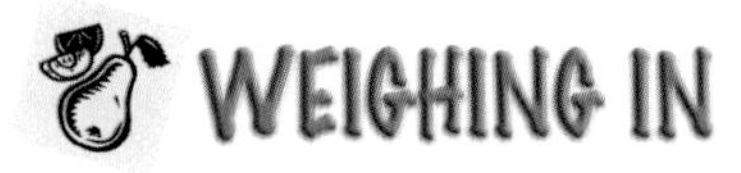

Healthy Weight Loss

- Set a goal to lose only 10 percent of your current weight to start with.
- Plan to lose about one-half to one pound (.5 kg) per week.
- Plateaus are normal.
- Keep a positive attitude!
- Emphasize eating fruits, vegetables, whole grains, and low-fat dairy products. Eat moderate amounts of fat and calories.

Setting a goal and working out a plan to reach it is important, but sometimes setting an impossible goal can get you into trouble. That's especially true when it comes to losing weight. Magazines trumpet miracle diets to help you lose weight fast. Drop 15 pounds in one week! Lose inches in a matter of days!

Don't believe it. The healthiest way to lose weight is gradually, and that means setting a reasonable goal, one that encourages, not discourages. Many experts say that if you're overweight, you should set a goal of losing 10 percent of your current weight. Let's say you weigh 180 pounds (81.6 kg). A reasonable goal would be to lose 18 pounds (8.2 kg) at a rate of about 1 pound (.5 kg) a week.

One pound a week means it won't happen overnight. Remember you're making a lifetime change. Don't be discouraged if you make a little progress then reach a plateau. That's perfectly normal, according to many weight-loss experts. Most people lose some weight, plateau, then lose a little more weight, especially if they increase their daily activity level.

If you are getting discouraged, examine your goals again and ask yourself if they are reasonable. If not, set a new goal, one you know you can reach. As long as you're staying active and eating a healthy diet that's got plenty of fruits, vegetables, whole grains, low-fat dairy products, and a limited amount of fat, especially saturated fat, then you're improving your health, whether you lose weight or not.

Just as there is no magic way to lose weight and keep it off, there is no miracle approach to staying active. Adopting an active lifestyle and sticking with it require commitment, planning, a positive outlook, and good old-fashioned perseverance. If you've learned one thing by sticking with our program, it's that you can make it happen. You can change for the better.

Chapter Checklist

Before you move on to the next week's activities, make sure you

- Took a few moments to identify stubborn negative thoughts and replaced them with positive messages
- Fine-tuned your plan for adding activity to your daily life
- Made specific plans for dealing with obstacles that may come along

We're almost done. Just one week to go. In the coming week, we'll review the key concepts we've explored along the way and talk about simple ways to stay motivated as you move onward.

WEEK **TWENTY**

Onward and Upward

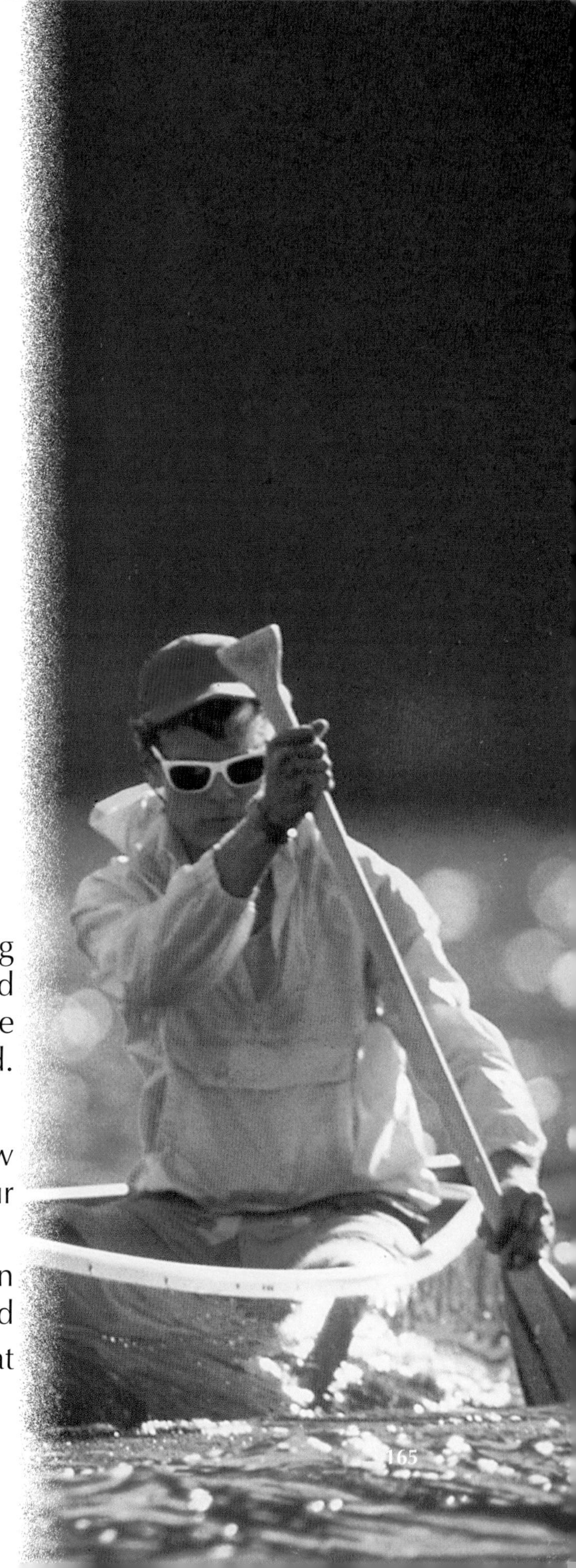

In This Chapter

- Reviewing key concepts
- Rating the skills and strategies that work best for you
- Making a commitment to the future

Let us be the first to congratulate you on reaching the end of this book. Chances are you've had some good times and some tough times along the way, and you've taken some giant steps forward. Specifically, we hope you've learned

- to think about physical activity in a new way—as something you can build into your everyday life,
- to incorporate short bouts of activity when you don't have time for longer sessions, and
- to monitor your activity and think about what support you need to stay active.

Most of all, we hope you've begun to think of yourself as an active person. Like many endings, in fact, this is really the beginning—the beginning of your active life. In this last week we'll look back at some ideas we've shared. Then we'll examine how these strategies can help you continue to improve. Finally, we're going to ask you to make a specific commitment over the next weeks and months to keep up the good work.

EXPERT ADVICE

What We've Learned

Our work at The Cooper Institute and Brown University, along with the work of many other scientists around the world, has demonstrated the remarkable benefits of an active lifestyle. We've also gained important insights into how people change behavior. That work has provided useful strategies to help people give up bad habits and adopt healthy ones, including changing an inactive lifestyle into an active way of life.

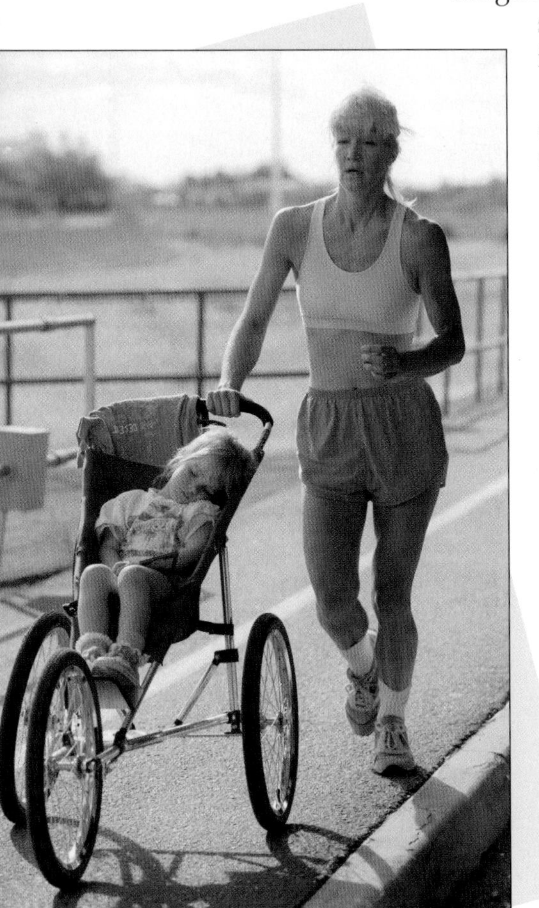

The more active you are, the bigger payoff you'll get.

Here's a quick checklist of the important insights we've explored over the past few months. Think about each one and how it applies to your experiences since you began:

- Strenuous exercise isn't the only way to reap the benefits of physical activity. Moderate-intensity activities such as brisk walking provide important health benefits.
- Thirty minutes of moderate-intensity activity every day can lower disease risk and help keep most people fit.
- Exercise doesn't have to be continuous. Short activities that add up to at least 30 minutes a day count.
- People's readiness to change varies from individual to individual.
- The process of change takes place in stages. For some people the process takes longer than for others.
- People who adopt skills such as setting short-term and long-term goals, recruiting support, rewarding themselves, and thinking positively are likely to maintain an active lifestyle over the long term.
- Everyone experiences setbacks on the path to change. People who eventually succeed learn to view setbacks as learning experiences.
- Planning how to meet your goal is essential to successful lifestyle change.
- Everyone encounters obstacles. One key to success is anticipating problems and having solutions prepared before they happen.
- Being physically active every day is a crucial part of losing weight and keeping it off.
- The more active you are the bigger the payoff in health, improved fitness, and a positive outlook.

ACTIVITY ALERT

What's Your Strategy?

Too often we don't take time to reflect on how far we've come. By charting our progress and distinguishing what's important from what's not, we can gain valuable lessons for the future.

Here's something else we've learned in our program: No single approach to lifestyle change works for everyone. Working with hundreds of people in our programs, we've seen that everyone is different. The people who made a lasting change were usually those who came to understand what worked for them. Understanding what makes *you* tick is the key to sticking with your program.

You guessed it: one more form to fill out. This is the last one—you've got our word on it. We think this one will be especially useful, as you set off on your own. The goal is to think critically about which skills and strategies worked best for *you*. Which strategies were important to your success? Which ones weren't important? Give yourself time to think about each one carefully.

WHAT WORKS, WHAT DOESN'T?

	Very important	Somewhat important	Not important
1. Replacing sedentary activities such as watching television with active ones such as taking short walks.			
2. Becoming aware of the benefits of being physically active.			
3. Setting short- and long-term goals for becoming and staying active.			
4. Rewarding myself for reaching my short- and long-term goals.			
5. Getting support from my family and friends.			
6. Understanding the benefits of physical activity that matter to me.			
7. Monitoring how much activity I do every day by counting steps or minutes.			
8. Becoming flexible in thinking about physical activities. For example, understanding that many types of activity count as exercise.			
9. Finding new opportunities for activity close to my work and home.			
10. Planning ahead for situations that might cause me to relapse.			

(continued)

(continued)

What other strategies have helped you along the way? List them here:

____

____

Look over your answers now, and circle the strategies that have made a difference for you. Keep them in mind whenever you hit a rocky stretch. They represent your personal keys to achieving success.

UP CLOSE & PERSONAL

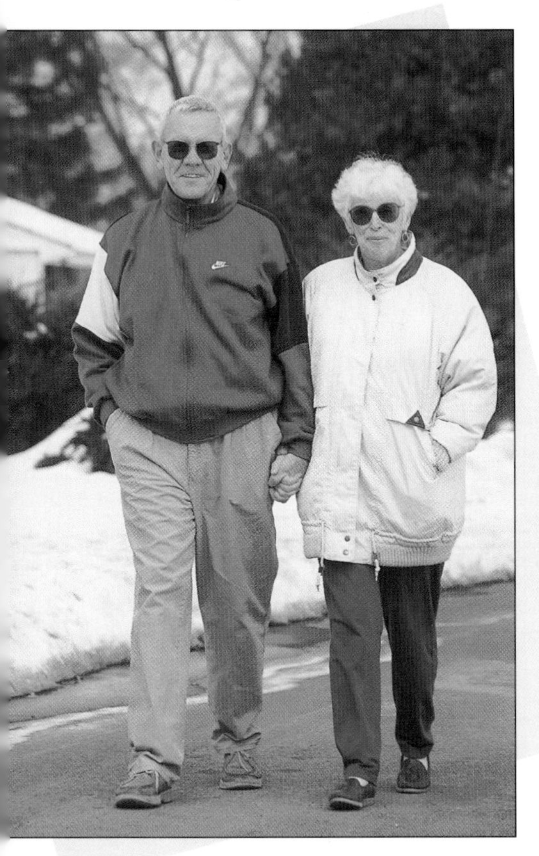

Like many people who have participated in our programs, Joyce knew she needed to increase her activity. She'd watched her mother's health decline and with it her ability to do simple things like climbing the stairs or loading the dishwasher. Joyce wanted to do what she could to make sure she would remain active as long as possible. She and her husband were already talking about retirement. Now she wanted to make sure she would be able to enjoy it.

At first, it wasn't easy. Joyce had to push herself hard to take even 10-minute walks. The only way she motivated herself was to think of them as a necessity. As she put it, "I'm not thrilled when I brush my teeth, but I wouldn't go a day without doing it! I realize this is something that I'm going to have to work at every day. I know when my husband and I retire, I want to be able to travel, to play with our grandchildren, and to know that I am able to continue doing all the things I enjoy."

A few months ago, six months after she finished the program, Joyce contacted us to say that she was staying active, even though she'd had a major relapse when her mother became ill and had to be hospitalized. "I started going through the workbook gradually again, and this time I learned some things I hadn't picked up on before. It helped to go back and think of what I had learned and why I wanted to be active."

Tips for Troubleshooting

Over time, many participants in our program returned to earlier weeks when they encountered trouble or needed a little encouragement. That's why we recommend that you keep this book handy, in case you need expert advice or a little nudge in the right direction. To help you find what you need, we've made a checklist of some common problems that arise for people as they move forward on the stages of change—and where to go for help.

- *Not enough time in the day to be active?* Look back to week 2 and complete a new Personal Time Study. The form will help you identify occasions when you can turn inactivity into activity.
- *Running into unexpected obstacles?* Look back at week 5 and the form called Great IDEA! It will help you identify barriers and formulate a plan to get past them.
- *Wondering how much energy you're expending?* Use the calorie calculation form in week 6 and the chart in appendix C to help you keep track of the number of calories you are burning in different physical activities.
- *Having trouble setting goals?* Week 7 is full of helpful hints for how to set reasonable and attainable goals that will motivate you to move forward.
- *Looking for support in your efforts to change?* Check out week 8, where you'll find useful advice about how to enlist the help you need from family and friends.
- *Sidelined by unexpected problems?* The activities in week 12 will help you identify and avoid common pitfalls.
- *Undone by too much stress?* Stress can undermine almost anyone's physical activity efforts. Week 13 offers simple ways to defuse even the most stressful situations.
- *Having trouble managing your time?* Check out the advice in week 15 on managing time and setting priorities.
- *Looking for a troubleshooting strategy that works best for you?* Return to your answers to the questionnaire on page 167 of this chapter.

Parting Words

The rest is up to you. You now have the tools and know-how to become active and make other healthy changes in your life. We hope you've also gained the self-confidence to know that you can make a change if you set your mind to it.

In the end, what you need to maintain the active lifestyle you've begun is exactly what you needed when you first opened this book: commitment. The only people who succeed at lifelong change are people who have committed themselves to learn the skills and strategies that make new habits stick.

So we'd like to ask you to do one more thing before you close the book. Think for a few moments about where you'd like to be three months from now. What kinds of activities would you like to be doing? How often? What barriers would you like to overcome? When you have your answer, take a piece of paper and write it down in the form of a commitment you make with yourself. It could be as simple as "Walk at least 45 minutes a day, five days a week," or "Stick to my goals through the coming holidays." It could be a resolution such as "Don't let negative thoughts get in my way, even when I'm stressed out," or perhaps something practical, such as "Join an indoor water aerobics class during the winter months," or "Encourage a few of my coworkers to become active this year." If you're feeling confident, write down two or three promises to yourself.

Now take the paper and tape it somewhere prominent—on your computer screen at work or the refrigerator door at home. This is your pledge to yourself. With your newfound confidence and skills, you can make it happen.

Making a lasting change in your life is something you have to work at, but it can be fun as well as rewarding. If this book has taught you one thing, we hope it's this: The effort it takes to become active is richly rewarded by the many benefits.

Keep up the good work!

APPENDIX A

Signs and Symptoms of Heart Attack and Stroke

If you or a loved one experiences any of these symptoms, call 911 or your local emergency number immediately. Treatment is often more effective if given quickly.

Heart Attack Warning Signs

- Pressure, fullness, squeezing, or crushing pain in the middle of the chest that lasts more than a few minutes, or goes away and comes back
- Pain that spreads to the shoulders, arms, back, neck, or jaw
- Lightheadedness, dizziness, or fainting
- Unexplained profuse or intense sweating
- Unusual stomach or abdominal pain
- Nausea or vomiting
- Shortness of breath and difficulty breathing
- Unexplained anxiety, sense of impending doom, weakness, or fatigue
- Palpitations, cold sweat, or paleness

Not every heart attack produces chest pain. Women usually experience the same pain and pressure (or other symptoms) as men do, but the tendency of women and their doctors is to ascribe it to something other than a heart attack. All people should take these symptoms seriously.

Stroke Warning Signs

- Sudden but often temporary numbness or weakness of the face, arm, or leg, especially on one side of the body

- Sudden language problems, such as slurred or difficult speech, or seeming to be confused
- Sudden visual disturbances, such as blocked or partial loss of vision in one or both eyes
- Abrupt and profound trouble walking, dizziness, loss of balance or coordination
- Sudden massive headache with no known cause

APPENDIX B

Stages on the Way to Becoming Active

Change doesn't happen overnight. Most people go through five stages on the way to making any kind of lasting change, whether it's becoming active, kicking the smoking habit, or adopting a new diet. These are the five stages of change involved in becoming active:

1. Not even thinking about it (precontemplation)
2. Giving it a thought now and then, but not doing it (comtemplation)
3. Doing it irregularly (preparation)
4. Doing the new habit consistently but for less than six months (action)
5. Maintaining the new habit for six months or more (maintenance)

Take a careful look at the five stages and identify where you are now. Be honest. In the following five sections, we'll help you identify strategies for moving ahead to the next stage and closer to the goal of becoming active. In our studies at Brown University, these strategies have helped people just like you to become more active.

Stage 1: Do I Need This?

Not Even Thinking About Being Active

If you are at stage 1, you haven't become convinced that being active is worth the effort. You don't have any plans to get up and get moving.

If you're like most people at stage 1, the list of reasons you have *not* to exercise is longer than the list of reasons why you want to increase your activity. Some reasons include the following:

- "I don't have time to increase my activity."
- "I don't like to exercise."
- "I tried in the past and I didn't get anything but sore muscles."
- "I'm too tired to exercise."

We'd like to convince you that you can overcome these reasons. We'd also like to persuade you that there are more good reasons to become active than to stay inactive. These include the following:

Material from copyrighted manuals (*Do I Need This?*; *Try It, You'll Like It*; *I'm on My Way*; *Keep It Going*; and *I Won't Stop Now*), developed by Bess H. Marcus, PhD, and colleagues of the Miriam Hospital, Providence, RI, has been adapted with permission. For more information, contact **LSExercise@lifespan.org** or call 401-793-3729.

- Activity can be fun.
- It's good for you.
- Physical activity can improve your blood cholesterol level.
- Moderate-intensity activity can reduce or even prevent high blood pressure.
- Physical activity helps in preventing and treating diabetes.
- Adding everyday activity can help you maintain a healthy weight.
- Physical activity is a great stress reliever.
- Regular exercise can decrease feelings of sadness and depression.

ACTIVITY ALERT

Think about the barriers and benefits of physical activity, using the following questions. Start with the barriers. What do you think?

1	2	3	4	5
Disagree strongly	Disagree somewhat	Neutral	Agree somewhat	Agree strongly

	1	2	3	4	5
1. Regular exercise would take too much of my time.					
2. At the end of the day I am much too tired to exercise.					
3. I would have less time for my family and friends if I exercised regularly.					
Add your answers to the last 3 questions: TOTAL [________________]					
This is your *barriers* score.					

Now think about some positive statements about physical activity:

	1	2	3	4	5
1. I would feel better about myself if I became active.					
2. I would feel less stressed if I exercised regularly.					
3. I would feel more comfortable with my body if I became active.					
Add your answers to the last 3 questions: TOTAL [________________]					
This is your *benefits* score.					

Which score is higher—the barriers or the benefits?

If you scored higher on benefits, that means you're becoming convinced that being active is important enough to make the effort. To move yourself forward, talk to friends or family members who make activity a regular part of their lives. Ask them what they do and what benefits they gain. Ask for their advice about simple ways to get started.

If your barriers score was higher, take time this week to list all the good things you can think of about an active lifestyle. What benefits of activity would be most important to you? Also think about the reasons you have for not being more active than you are now. Begin to think about ways you might work around them.

Stage 2: Try It, You'll Like It

Giving It a Thought Now and Then, but Not Doing It

If you're at stage 2 on the path to an active life, you're already thinking seriously about becoming active. That's great. Now is the time to consider ways to turn that good intention into action.

ACTIVITY ALERT

Use the four Ws to begin planning for activity. Circle your answer for each question, or add an answer of your own.

What activity would you be willing to try?
(Think about things you've enjoyed doing in the past or activities that look like fun.)

Walking Gardening Bicycling Swimming Dancing Other

When could you find 10 minutes to be active?

In the morning At lunch After work After dinner Other

Where is the best place for you to be active?

At home In the neighborhood At the YMCA Other

Who do you want to be active with?

Just myself Friends from work
My spouse or partner My family Other

Use your answers to begin to create a plan. If you want to try walking and morning is the best time for you, schedule a time this week to try it. Encourage your spouse or partner to join you if you prefer to have company, or strike out on your own if you'd rather go solo. Enjoy yourself!

Stage 3: On My Way

Doing It Irregularly

If you're at stage 3, you are active now and then, but you haven't been able to make a regular habit of it. Don't be discouraged. You're already well on the way. Now is the time to think about ways to encourage yourself to become regularly active.

ACTIVITY ALERT

Start by thinking about times recently when you have become inactive for too long. What happened? What obstacles got in your way? List a few of the most difficult hurdles you faced:

Obstacle 1 ______________________________

____

Obstacle 2 ______________________________

____

Obstacle 3 ______________________________

____

Now brainstorm solutions to these obstacles. Here are some suggestions:

- If you find it hard to remember to exercise, put a note on your calendar at work to remind yourself. Leave your walking shoes by the door at home as a reminder.
- If you become inactive when the weather is bad, develop a backup plan. You can walk at the mall on rainy days, for instance. If you live where the winters are long and cold, look into buying an exercise cycle.
- If you stopped exercising because you weren't in the mood, remember that activity improves people's moods. It not only relieves stress but also helps fight sadness and depression. Push yourself to get up and get moving, even if you're in a bad mood. Doing a little is better than doing nothing.

Look back at your list of obstacles and write down at least one possible solution. The next time you find yourself falling off the activity bandwagon, use these ideas to help get back on track.▌

Remember to reward yourself often for a job well done. Set a goal of being active almost every day for the next two weeks. If you do so, celebrate by treating yourself to something special.

Stage 4: Sticking to It

Doing the New Habit Consistently but for Less Than Six Months

If you're at stage 4, you are active almost every day, but you haven't managed yet to get beyond the six-month mark. No problem. There are simple strategies that will help you turn activity into a lifelong habit.

Set goals. This is one of the best ways to stay focused and motivated. Think about what you want to accomplish over the next month. Then decide what you need to do to get there. Make your goal simple and reasonable enough that you can reach it. Then break the work down into small, easy tasks. Each task is a short-term goal. As you perform each short-term goal, you will move another step toward your long-term goal. Remember to reward yourself when you accomplish your goals.

Try different activities. One obstacle many people face is boredom. After a while, the thrill of walking through the same neighborhood streets begins to wear off. Swimming is wonderful exercise, but every once in a while it's fun to try something else. If you'd rather not change your activities, at least change the setting. Discover a new neighborhood to walk or bicycle in. Try a different swimming stroke, or join a water aerobics class. Another way to prevent your activity routine from becoming boring is to exercise with a friend.

Think about your past successes. By this time, you've had plenty of good weeks when you've been active almost every day. You've also had some weeks when it has been hard for you to overcome the obstacles to exercising. What methods did you use to get past those hurdles? How did it feel to reach your short-term goals? Remind yourself that you can make it if you try.

Choose a role model. One way to motivate yourself is to find someone you look up to—someone at work or in the family who has made exercise a lifelong habit. Sit down and tell this person about your goal to increase your activity. Ask for advice. If you don't have someone close to talk to, consider joining a club that offers your favorite activity. You may make a few friends who will motivate you. Along the way, you'll be able to give them a little extra push as well.

Stage 5: I'm on Track

Maintaining the New Habit for Six Months or More

If you're at stage 5, you have been active almost every day for six months or more. Congratulations. You're well on your way to making activity a lifelong habit.

This book is full of advice to help you overcome any obstacles you may encounter. Keep it handy just in case you need help along the way. With a long record of success behind you, you can feel confident that you can make it if you stay focused on your goal of staying active.

If you find yourself becoming inactive for a week or a couple weeks, it's important to understand why and push yourself to get up and get moving. Otherwise you could lose the exercise habit. If this happens to you, make a plan to become active as soon as possible. Set a date and choose a specific activity. Once you've taken one walk or participated in one aerobics class, the next ones will be easier.

Now that you've proven you can do it, take time to encourage a friend or family member to become active. Be a mentor, and you'll find new reasons to stay active yourself.

ACTIVITY ALERT

To be ready for any obstacles that may come along, take a few minutes to answer some questions.

1. Have you ever stopped being active for a week or more in the past?

   ____

   ____

   ____

2. What caused you to stop?

   ____

   ____

   ____

3. What did you do to get started again?

   ____

   ____

   ____

4. What obstacles are likely to be a problem for you now?

   ____

   ____

   ____

5. What can you do to prepare for those obstacles?

   ____

   ____

   ____

6. What will help you get back on track if you stop being active?

   ____

   ____

   ____

If you run into trouble in the future, look back at your answers. They could encourage you to get moving again. Meanwhile, keep up the good work, and enjoy the many benefits of an active life!

APPENDIX C

Energy Expenditure Chart

Estimated calories burned per minute of activity

	kg	55	64	73	82	91	100	109	118	127
ACTIVITIES	**lb**	120	140	160	180	200	220	240	260	280
Light										
Child care, sitting or kneeling		2.4	2.8	3.2	3.6	4.0	4.4	4.8	5.2	5.6
Cleaning sink, tub, or toilet		2.4	2.8	3.2	3.6	4.0	4.4	4.8	5.2	5.6
Cleaning, light (dusting, picking up)		2.4	2.8	3.2	3.6	4.0	4.4	4.8	5.2	5.6
Cooking		1.9	2.2	2.6	2.9	3.2	3.5	3.8	4.1	4.4
Fishing, boat		2.4	2.8	3.2	3.6	4.0	4.4	4.8	5.2	5.6
Fishing, ice		1.9	2.2	2.6	2.9	3.2	3.5	3.8	4.1	4.4
Hand sewing		1.9	2.2	2.6	2.9	3.2	3.5	3.8	4.1	4.4
Horseback riding at a walk		2.4	2.8	3.2	3.6	4.0	4.4	4.8	5.2	5.6
Ironing		2.2	2.6	2.9	3.3	3.7	4.0	4.4	4.7	5.1
Mowing lawn, riding mower		2.4	2.8	3.2	3.6	4.0	4.4	4.8	5.2	5.6
Pistol or trap shooting		2.4	2.8	3.2	3.6	4.0	4.4	4.8	5.2	5.6
Playing catch		2.4	2.8	3.2	3.6	4.0	4.4	4.8	5.2	5.6
Playing croquet		2.4	2.8	3.2	3.6	4.0	4.4	4.8	5.2	5.6
Playing pool		2.4	2.8	3.2	3.6	4.0	4.4	4.8	5.2	5.6
Shopping		2.2	2.6	2.9	3.3	3.7	4.0	4.4	4.7	5.1
Sitting, playing cards, at sporting event, in meetings		1.4	1.7	1.9	2.2	2.4	2.6	2.9	3.1	3.3
Sitting, typing or writing		1.7	2.0	2.3	2.6	2.9	3.2	3.4	3.7	4.0
Sleeping		0.9	1.0	1.1	1.3	1.4	1.6	1.7	1.9	2.0
Standing		1.7	2.0	2.3	2.6	2.9	3.2	3.4	3.7	4.0
Stretching		2.4	2.8	3.2	3.6	4.0	4.4	4.8	5.2	5.6
Walking, 30 min per mile (1.6 km)		2.4	2.8	3.2	3.6	4.0	4.4	4.8	5.2	5.6
Washing dishes, standing		2.2	2.6	2.9	3.3	3.7	4.0	4.4	4.7	5.1
Watching TV, sitting or lying		1.0	1.1	1.3	1.4	1.6	1.8	1.9	2.1	2.2

(continued)

(continued)

ACTIVITIES	kg lb	55 120	64 140	73 160	82 180	91 200	100 220	109 240	118 260	127 280
		Estimated calories burned per minute of activity								
Moderate										
Aerobic dance, low impact		4.8	5.6	6.4	7.2	8.0	8.8	9.5	10.3	11.1
Archery		3.4	3.9	4.5	5.0	5.6	6.1	6.7	7.2	7.8
Badminton		4.3	5.0	5.7	6.5	7.2	7.9	8.6	9.3	10.0
Bicycling, 10 mph		3.9	4.5	5.1	5.7	6.4	7.0	7.6	8.3	8.9
Bowling		2.9	3.4	3.8	4.3	4.8	5.3	5.7	6.2	6.7
Canoeing		3.9	4.5	5.1	5.7	6.4	7.0	7.6	8.3	8.9
Carpentry, general		2.9	3.4	3.8	4.3	4.8	5.3	5.7	6.2	6.7
Carrying small children		2.9	3.4	3.8	4.3	4.8	5.3	5.7	6.2	6.7
Dancing, line, polka, country		4.3	5.0	5.7	6.5	7.2	7.9	8.6	9.3	10.0
Dancing, waltz, foxtrot, samba		2.9	3.4	3.8	4.3	4.8	5.3	5.7	6.2	6.7
Fishing, from bank		3.4	3.9	4.5	5.0	5.6	6.1	6.7	7.2	7.8
Kayaking		4.8	5.6	6.4	7.2	8.0	8.8	9.5	10.3	11.1
Laying sod		4.8	5.6	6.4	7.2	8.0	8.8	9.5	10.3	11.1
Mopping, vacuuming		3.4	3.9	4.5	5.0	5.6	6.1	6.7	7.2	7.8
Mowing lawn, power mower		4.3	5.0	5.7	6.5	7.2	7.9	8.6	9.3	10.0
Painting, exterior		4.8	5.6	6.4	7.2	8.0	8.8	9.5	10.3	11.1
Painting, interior		2.9	3.4	3.8	4.3	4.8	5.3	5.7	6.2	6.7
Playing Frisbee, light		2.9	3.4	3.8	4.3	4.8	5.3	5.7	6.2	6.7
Playing golf, no cart		4.3	5.0	5.7	6.5	7.2	7.9	8.6	9.3	10.0
Playing in marching band		3.9	4.5	5.1	5.7	6.4	7.0	7.6	8.3	8.9
Playing shuffleboard		2.9	3.4	3.8	4.3	4.8	5.3	5.7	6.2	6.7
Playing softball		4.8	5.6	6.4	7.2	8.0	8.8	9.5	10.3	11.1
Raking lawn		3.9	4.5	5.1	5.7	6.4	7.0	7.6	8.3	8.9
Skateboarding		4.8	5.6	6.4	7.2	8.0	8.8	9.5	10.3	11.1
Snorkeling		4.8	5.6	6.4	7.2	8.0	8.8	9.5	10.3	11.1
Snowmobiling		3.4	3.9	4.5	5.0	5.6	6.1	6.7	7.2	7.8
Sweeping sidewalk		3.9	4.5	5.1	5.7	6.4	7.0	7.6	8.3	8.9
Swimming, treading water		3.9	4.5	5.1	5.7	6.4	7.0	7.6	8.3	8.9
Table tennis		3.9	4.5	5.1	5.7	6.4	7.0	7.6	8.3	8.9
Tai chi		3.9	4.5	5.1	5.7	6.4	7.0	7.6	8.3	8.9
Trampoline		3.4	3.9	4.5	5.0	5.6	6.1	6.7	7.2	7.8
Trimming shrubs, manual clipper		4.3	5.0	5.7	6.5	7.2	7.9	8.6	9.3	10.0
Walking, 15 min per mile (1.6 km)		4.8	5.6	6.4	7.2	8.0	8.8	9.5	10.3	11.1
Walking, 20 min per mile (1.6 km)		3.2	3.7	4.2	4.7	5.3	5.8	6.3	6.8	7.3
Washing and waxing automobile		2.9	3.4	3.8	4.3	4.8	5.3	5.7	6.2	6.7
Water aerobics		3.9	4.5	5.1	5.7	6.4	7.0	7.6	8.3	8.9
Weeding, digging in garden		4.3	5.0	5.7	6.5	7.2	7.9	8.6	9.3	10.0
Hard										
Aerobic dance, high impact		6.7	7.8	8.9	10.0	11.1	12.3	13.4	14.5	15.6
Carpentry (e.g., fence building, roofing)		5.8	6.7	7.7	8.6	9.6	10.5	11.4	12.4	13.3

ACTIVITIES	kg / lb	55 / 120	64 / 140	73 / 160	82 / 180	91 / 200	100 / 220	109 / 240	118 / 260	127 / 280
Chopping wood		5.8	6.7	7.7	8.6	9.6	10.5	11.4	12.4	13.3
Circuit training		7.7	9.0	10.2	11.5	12.7	14.0	15.3	16.5	17.8
Fishing, wading in stream		5.8	6.7	7.7	8.6	9.6	10.5	11.4	12.4	13.3
Horseback riding at trot		6.3	7.3	8.3	9.3	10.4	11.4	12.4	13.4	14.4
Marching, race walking		6.3	7.3	8.3	9.3	10.4	11.4	12.4	13.4	14.4
Moving furniture		5.8	6.7	7.7	8.6	9.6	10.5	11.4	12.4	13.3
Mowing lawn, hand mower		5.8	6.7	7.7	8.6	9.6	10.5	11.4	12.4	13.3
Playing tennis, doubles		5.8	6.7	7.7	8.6	9.6	10.5	11.4	12.4	13.3
Playing racquetball, casual		6.7	7.8	8.9	10.0	11.1	12.3	13.4	14.5	15.6
Rowing, moderate effort		6.7	7.8	8.9	10.0	11.1	12.3	13.4	14.5	15.6
Sawing wood by hand		6.7	7.8	8.9	10.0	11.1	12.3	13.4	14.5	15.6
Shoveling, light to moderate		6.3	7.3	8.3	9.3	10.4	11.4	12.4	13.4	14.4
Skating, roller or ice		6.7	7.8	8.9	10.0	11.1	12.3	13.4	14.5	15.6
Ski machine		6.7	7.8	8.9	10.0	11.1	12.3	13.4	14.5	15.6
Skiing, downhill, moderate effort		5.8	6.7	7.7	8.6	9.6	10.5	11.4	12.4	13.3
Skin diving		6.7	7.8	8.9	10.0	11.1	12.3	13.4	14.5	15.6
Swimming, lap, light/moderate effort		6.7	7.8	8.9	10.0	11.1	12.3	13.4	14.5	15.6
Swimming, leisure		5.8	6.7	7.7	8.6	9.6	10.5	11.4	12.4	13.3
Walking with a backpack		6.7	7.8	8.9	10.0	11.1	12.3	13.4	14.5	15.6
Weightlifting, vigorous effort		5.8	6.7	7.7	8.6	9.6	10.5	11.4	12.4	13.3
Very hard										
Bicycling, 12-14 mph		7.7	9.0	10.2	11.5	12.7	14.0	15.3	16.5	17.8
Bicycling, 16-19 mph		11.6	13.4	15.3	17.2	19.1	21.0	22.9	24.8	26.7
Canoeing, vigorous effort		11.6	13.4	15.3	17.2	19.1	21.0	22.9	24.8	26.7
Cross-country skiing		8.7	10.1	11.5	12.9	14.3	15.8	17.2	18.6	20.0
Digging ditches		8.2	9.5	10.9	12.2	13.5	14.9	16.2	17.6	18.9
Horseback riding, galloping		7.7	9.0	10.2	11.5	12.7	14.0	15.3	16.5	17.8
In-line skating		12.0	14.0	16.0	17.9	19.9	21.9	23.8	25.8	27.8
Judo, karate, kick boxing		9.6	11.2	12.8	14.4	15.9	17.5	19.1	20.7	22.2
Mountain biking		8.2	9.5	10.9	12.2	13.5	14.9	16.2	17.6	18.9
Playing basketball		7.7	9.0	10.2	11.5	12.7	14.0	15.3	16.5	17.8
Playing football		7.7	9.0	10.2	11.5	12.7	14.0	15.3	16.5	17.8
Playing handball		11.6	13.4	15.3	17.2	19.1	21.0	22.9	24.8	26.7
Playing hockey, field or ice		7.7	9.0	10.2	11.5	12.7	14.0	15.3	16.5	17.8
Playing racquetball, competitive		9.6	11.2	12.8	14.4	15.9	17.5	19.1	20.7	22.2
Playing tennis, singles		7.7	9.0	10.2	11.5	12.7	14.0	15.3	16.5	17.8
Playing soccer		9.6	11.2	12.8	14.4	15.9	17.5	19.1	20.7	22.2
Playing volleyball		7.7	9.0	10.2	11.5	12.7	14.0	15.3	16.5	17.8
Rowing, vigorous effort		11.6	13.4	15.3	17.2	19.1	21.0	22.9	24.8	26.7
Running, 8 min per mile (1.6 km)		12.0	14.0	16.0	17.9	19.9	21.9	23.8	25.8	27.8
Running, 10 min per mile		9.6	11.2	12.8	14.4	15.9	17.5	19.1	20.7	22.2

(continued)

(continued)

Estimated calories burned per minute of activity

ACTIVITIES	kg lb	55 120	64 140	73 160	82 180	91 200	100 220	109 240	118 260	127 280
Skipping rope		7.7	9.0	10.2	11.5	12.7	14.0	15.3	16.5	17.8
Snow shoeing		10.6	12.3	14.1	15.8	17.5	19.3	21.0	22.7	24.4
Stair climber machine		8.7	10.1	11.5	12.9	14.3	15.8	17.2	18.6	20.0
Step aerobics, 6- to 8-in. step		8.2	9.5	10.9	12.2	13.5	14.9	16.2	17.6	18.9
Swimming, vigorous effort		10.6	12.3	14.1	15.8	17.5	19.3	21.0	22.7	24.4
Walking, 12 min per mile (1.6 km)		7.7	9.0	10.2	11.5	12.7	14.0	15.3	16.5	17.8

Based on selected MET values created by B.E. Ainsworth, W.L. Haskell, M.C. Whitt, M.L. Irwin, A.M. Swartz, et al., 2000, "Compendium of physical activities: An update of activity codes and MET intensities." *Medicine and Science in Sports and Exercise* 32 (9): S498-504.

APPENDIX D

Forms: Progressing Toward an Active Lifestyle

PERSONAL TIME STUDY

Date: ____________________ Day of week: ______________________

Time slot	Tasks/activities	Physically active? Yes	No
Midnight to 4:00 A.M.			
4:01 to 8:00 A.M.			
8:01 A.M. to noon			
12:01 to 4:00 P.M.			
4:01 to 8:00 P.M.			
8:01 P.M. to midnight			
	Total time		

KEEPING TRACK OF THOUGHTS

Week of ______________________________

Instructions: Use this form to record the number of times you think about doing physical activity. Simply place a check mark (✔) in a box in section 1 each time you *think* about doing some physical activity. If you carried out your thoughts and did the activity you were thinking about, place a check mark (✔) in a box in section 2.

Keeping track of your thoughts about activity can help you start moving toward an active lifestyle.

Section 1 I thought about doing some physical activity.

Section 2 I carried out my thoughts and did the activity.

KEEPING TRACK OF PHYSICAL ACTIVITY

Activity minutes	Intensity level	2 minutes	10 minutes	Total minutes
Garden	Moderate			
	Vigorous			
Household	Moderate			
	Vigorous			
Leisure	Moderate			
	Vigorous			
Occupation	Moderate			
	Vigorous			
Sports	Moderate			
	Vigorous			
Stairs	Moderate (1 flight up = 10 steps)			
	Vigorous (4 flights up = 2 minutes vigorous work)			
Walking	Moderate			
	Vigorous			

STEP-BY-STEP

WEEKLY ACTIVITY LOG

Week: ______________________

Day of week	Date	Step goal	Actual steps	Minutes of activity Moderate	Hard	Notes
Monday						
Tuesday						
Wednesday						
Thursday						
Friday						
Saturday						
Sunday						

Week: ______________________

Day of week	Date	Step goal	Actual steps	Minutes of activity Moderate	Hard	Notes
Monday						
Tuesday						
Wednesday						
Thursday						
Friday						
Saturday						
Sunday						

REFERENCES

1. James WPT. 1995. A public health approach to the problem of obesity. *International Journal of Obesity and Related Metabolic Disorders.* 19(Suppl 3):S37-S45.
2. Dunn AL, Marcus BH, Kampert JB, Garcia ME, Kohl HW, Blair SN. 1999. Comparison of lifestyle and structured interventions to increase physical activity and cardiorespiratory fitness: a randomized trial. *Journal of the American Medical Association.* 281(4):327-334.
3. Jakicic JM, Wing RR, Butler BA, Robertson RJ. 1995. Prescribing exercise in multiple short bouts versus one continuous bout: effects on adherence, cardiorespiratory fitness, and weight loss in overweight women.. *International Journal of Obesity and Related Metabolic Disorders.* 19(12):893-901.
4. Neiman DC, Henson DA, Guswitch G, Warren BJ, Dotson RC, Butterworth DE, Nehlsen-Cannarella SL. 1993. Physical activity and immune function in elderly women. *Medicine and Science in Sports and Exercise.* 25(7):823-831.
5. Giovannucci E, Ascherio A, Rimm EB, Colditz GA, Stampfer MJ, Willett WC. 1995. Physical activity, obesity and risk of colon cancer and adenoma in men. *Annals of Internal Medicine.* 122(5):327-334.
6. Brownell KD, Stunkard AJ, Albaum JM. 1980. Evaluation and modification of exercise patterns in the natural environment. *American Journal of Psychiatry.* 137(12):1540-1545.
7. Boreham CA, Wallace WF, Nevill A. 2000. Training effects of accumulated daily stair-climbing exercise in previously sedentary young women. *Preventive Medicine.* 30(4):277-281.
8. Blair SN, Kampert JB, Kohl HW, Barlow CE, Macera CA, Paffenbarger RS, Gibbons LW. 1996. Influences of cardiorespiratory fitness and other precursors on cardiovascular disease and all-cause mortality in men and women. *Journal of the American Medical Association.* 276(3):205-210.
9. President's Council on Physical Fitness and Sports and the Sporting Goods Manufacturers Association. 1993. American attitudes toward physical activity and fitness: a national survey. A survey conducted by Peter D. Hart Research Associates, Washington DC.
10. Wei M, Gibbons LW, Kampert JB, Nichaman MZ, Blair SN. 2000. Low cardiorespiratory fitness and physical inactivity as predictors of mortality in men with type 2 diabetes. *Annals of Internal Medicine.* 132(8):605-611.
11. Hu FB, Sigal RJ, Rich-Edwards JW, Colditz GA, Solomon CG, Willett WC, Speizer FE, Manson JE. 1999. Walking compared with vigorous physical activity and risk of type 2 diabetes in women: a prospective study. *Journal of the American Medical Association.* 282(15):1433-1439.
12. Thune I. 1996. Physical activity and risk of colorectal cancer in men and women. *British Journal of Cancer.* 73(9):1134-1140.
13. Yanovski JA, Yanovski SZ, Sovik KN, Nguyen TT, O'Neil PM, Sebring NG. 2000. A prospective study of holiday weight gain. *New England Journal of Medicine.* 342(12):861-867.
14. Marcus BH, Albrecht AE, King TK, Parisi AF, Pinto B, Roberts M, Niaura RS, Abrams DB. 1999. The efficacy of exercise as an aid to smoking cessation in women: a randomized controlled trial. *Archives of Internal Medicine.* 159(11):1229-1234.
15. Berk LS, Tan SA, Fry WF, Napier BJ, Lee JW, Hubbard RW, Lewis JE, Eby WC. 1989. Neuroendocrine and stress hormone changes during mirthful laughter. *American Journal of Medicine and Science.* 298(6):390-396.
16. Lee DL, Blair SN, Jackson AS. 1999. Cardiorespiratory fitness, body composition, and all-cause and cardiovascular disease mortality in men. *American Journal of Clinical Nutrition.* 69(3):373-380.
17. Jakicic JM, Winters C, Lang W, Wing RR. 1999. Effects of intermittent exercise and use of home exercise equipment on adherence, weight loss, and fitness in overweight women: a randomized trial. *Journal of the American Medical Association.* 282(16):1554-1560.
18. Esparza J, Fox C, Harper IT, Bennett PH, Schulz LO, Valencia ME, Ravussin E. 2000. Daily energy expenditure in Mexican and USA Pima Indians: low physical activity as a possible cause of obesity. *International Journal of Obesity and Related Disorders.* 24(1):55-59.

INDEX